£6-25

PRENTICE-HALL

FOUNDATIONS OF IMMUNOLOGY SERIES

Abraham Osler and Leon Weiss, Editors

THE IMMUNOBIOLOGY OF TRANSPLANTATION
Rupert Billingham and Willys Silvers

THE CELLS AND TISSUES OF THE IMMUNE SYSTEM
Leon Weiss

IMMUNOCYTOCHEMISTRY
Ludwig A. Sternberger

IMMUNOCYTOCHEMISTRY

LUDWIG A. STERNBERGER

Edgewood Arsenal
and
The Johns Hopkins University School of Medicine

PRENTICE-HALL, INC., *Englewood Cliffs, N. J.*

Library of Congress Cataloging in Publication Data

STERNBERGER, LUDWIG A
   Immunocytochemistry.

   (Foundations of immunology series)
   Includes bibliographies.
   1. Immunochemistry. 2. Cytochemistry.
I. Title. DNLM: 1. Histocytochemistry.
2. Immunochemistry. QW504 S84li 1974
QR182.S7   574.2′9   73-14792
ISBN 0-13-451658-3

10 9 8 7 6 5 4 3 2 1

PRINTED IN THE UNITED STATES OF AMERICA

PRENTICE-HALL INTERNATIONAL, INC., *London*
PRENTICE-HALL OF AUSTRALIA, PTY. LTD., *Sydney*
PRENTICE-HALL OF CANADA, LTD., *Toronto*
PRENTICE-HALL OF INDIA PRIVATE LIMITED, *New Delhi*
PRENTICE-HALL OF JAPAN, INC., *Tokyo*

Foundations of Immunology Series

This series of monographs is intended to provide readers of diverse backgrounds with an authoritative and clear statement concerning significant aspects of immunology. Each volume represents an individual contribution by a distinguished scientist. As a series, they provide a comprehensive view of the field.

The editors have encouraged the individuality of each author in content and method of presentation. They have sought as the major objective of the series, that each monograph be comprehensible and of interest to a broad audience. The authors provide an authoritative treatment of important problems in major research areas, in which rapid development of new information requires an integrated and reliable evaluation. The series should therefore prove valuable to advanced college students, graduate students, medical students and house staff, practitioners of medicine, laboratory scientists, and teachers.

ABRAHAM OSLER
LEON WEISS

Contents

Preface

Immunocytochemistry is the study by immunologic methods of the nature of light and electron-microscopically observed cellular structure. Immunologic reagents are the tools that confer specificity to this analysis. The present book has been written for the biologist and pathologist seeking information on immunologic and immunocytochemical principles and for the immunologist interested in problems of cytology and pathology. The core of the book deals with the chemical and immunologic foundations of the various immunocytochemical methods and with the principles and scope of their applications. Procedural details are included to the extent of permitting the reader to apply the methods without necessarily referring to their original documentation. Applications of the methods are discussed with emphasis on specificities and sensitivities with the hope that a researcher can choose the particular method most suitable for his purpose.

Modern immunologic principles are outlined in sufficient detail that no previous knowledge of immunology is necessary. Most of the fundamental immunologic concepts are briefly discussed in the first chapter on immunoglobulin structure. Most of the applications to cellular immunology and immunopathology are in the concluding chapters. Historical approaches have usually been omitted in order to attain conciseness for the casual reader and information density for the researcher. Brevity also precluded complete literature coverage. However, I hope that the articles quoted in turn provide references that complete the bibliography.

Ludwig A. Sternberger

Chapter 1

Immunoglobulin Structure

Immunoglobulins are a diverse group of proteins defined by the specificity of their antibody function. They made their appearance rather late in evolution and have assumed importance for survival only in more recent forms of vertebrates. The specific reactivity of antibodies has extended the scope of immunoglobulins beyond their role in etiology, pathology, or diagnosis of most diseases. As the range of specificities within the capability of an individual is an inborn property, immunoglobulins are phenotypic expressions with which genetic endowment can be explored. The function of genetic predestination is limited to determining whether or not a host will respond to a specific, *antigenic stimulus*. Genetically given specificity does not, however, determine which pathway the response to a stimulus will take. Thus, the immune response permits for the first time dissection of the relative contributions of genetic and environmental factors in the response of an individual to extraneous stimuli.

The specificity of antibodies also suggests the use of immunoglobulins as reagents in the laboratory in applications that go beyond their biologic function. These applications are aided by the relative ease with which methods for the study of immunoglobulins can be developed. If we are interested in a neurotransmitter enzyme, such as acetylcholinesterase, we must contend with the amount of enzyme available in the synaptic tissue under investigation. On the other hand, if we are interested in an immunoglobulin, as for instance an immunoglobulin with antibody activity specific for corticotropin (anticorticotropin), we can by immunization induce replication of specific cells so that a preexisting minimal amount of anticorticotropin specificity on the surface of a few cells becomes amplified until large quantities of anticorticotropin are secreted by many cells. Although in our cholinesterase example the synaptic junction contains not only acetylcholinesterase but also variable amounts of acyl cholinesterase and nonspecific esterase, we can with immunoglobulins control the specificity of antibodies produced: for instance, we can induce antibodies to the peptides consisting of amino acids 17–39 of corticotropin, thus, obtain-

1

ing antibodies specific for corticotropin only and lacking specificity for the chemically related melanocyte-stimulating hormone often found in the same cell as corticotropin. The possibility of producing immunoglobulins at will in large quantities and controlling the specificity of their reaction expands the significance of antibodies from their role in biologic function (immunity, hypersensitivity, and possible control mechanisms) to that of biologic reagents. The use of antibodies as specific reagents for tissue constituents *in situ* is the domain of *immunocytochemistry*. Its success lies in the high specific selectivity of binding of antibodies induced during immunization by a specific *antigenic determinant* on the immunizing antigen.

The specificity of antibodies is due to selection during immunization of types of immunoglobulin that contain in their specific *combining sites* unique amino acid sequences that provide high binding affinity (*avidity*) for the antigenic determinant. This selection is possible because of pre-existence of a large number of differently structured specific combining sites: the combining site of immunoglobulins is in the *variable region* of the immunoglobulin molecule; that is, among different clones of immuno-competent cells, each produces immunoglobulins of a characteristic amino acid sequence in this region. The number of different antigenic determinants to which a host can respond is immense as is the number of types of immunocompetent cells he possesses. When immunoglobulin binds with a specific antigenic determinant, probably only some of the amino acids in the variable region come into direct contact. These amino acids undergo highest frequency variation from one random immunoglobulin molecule to another: their position in the immunoglobulin peptide structure defines the *hypervariable region*.

The variable region is the most characteristic part of the immuno-globulin molecule. Its function is essential for the specificity of the immunocytochemical reaction. The remainder of the immunoglobulin molecule is necessary for molding its individual peptides into a structural unit and for the secondary functions of antibodies before or after reaction with antigen in or on a cell or in circulation. These secondary functions include transport of immunoglobulin, immune elimination of antigen, and cyto-toxicity. The secondary functions often provide mechanisms that explain observations obtained from staining pathologic tissue with immunocyto-chemical methods. The structural features in immunoglobulin that contribute to the secondary functions are also utilized extensively in the development of the various immunocytochemical methods we will discuss in the following pages. The secondary functions reside in relatively *constant* amino acid sequences of the immunoglobulin molecule. Antibodies of different specificities may share identical amino acid sequences in the constant region. The nature of the constant region sequence determines the kind of secondary functions an immunoglobulin may undergo. The sequence does not contribute to specific binding. The term *constancy* of amino acid sequence only implies invariance of composition of immuno-globulins irrespective of their specificities for binding antigenic determi-nants. However, there do exist a great number of different constant region sequences that a vertebrate is capable of producing. While some of these variations determine unique secondary properties, others may be without specific biologic function. In general, the differences in amino acid com-position of the constant region that determine differences in secondary functions are extensive. The constant region is characteristic of the *class* to which an immunoglobulin molecule belongs. Different classes of im-munoglobulins are easy to separate. Minor differences within only few amino acids in the constant regions of immunoglobulin molecules within classes can be detected by more extensive separation methods. These vari-ations determine *subclasses* of immunoglobulins. Genetic markers specify the amino acid composition of definite *loci* in each peptide chain of im-munoglobulin molecules. These allelic markers (genetically paired, alter-native markers) are detected by reaction of the immunoglobulin as antigen with antiserum produced in allogenic hosts.

Even antibodies purified from a single subclass of immunoglobulin by reaction with a specific antigen are usually heterogeneous because of dif-ferences of conformation of the specific binding sites to different portions of a single antigenic determinant. These antibodies are, therefore, not suitable for studying the amino acid sequence of the specific combining sites. The homogeneous antibodies that have contributed so much to the elucidation of immunoglobulin structure are the product of clones of anti-body-producing cells derived from a single antigen-recognizing cell. These antibodies are provided in large quantities by monoclonal tumors of anti-body-producing cells (plasmacytomas, multiple myelomas) and in small quantities by the immediate environment of an individual antibody-produc-ing cell in culture on semisolid medium. Antibodies of restricted hetero-geneity are also obtained occasionally by purification from hyperimmune sera after immunization with antigens consisting of regularly repeated sequences of identical constituents, such as lipopolysaccharides or tobacco mosaic virus.

IMMUNOGLOBULIN G

The bulk of antibodies obtained after hyperimmunization with most antigens resides in the immunoglobulin G (IgG) class. At pH 8.6 IgG possesses the slowest electrophoretic mobility among serum proteins. This property and its low solubility at low ionic strength facilitates its con-venient isolation by passage through a diethylaminoethyl cellulose column at pH 6.5–8.0 in 0.005–0.02 M phosphate buffer. Under these conditions

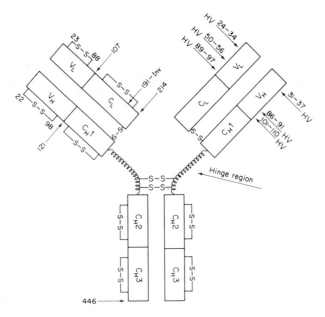

Fig. 1-1 The complete amino acid sequence of a myeloma immunoglobulin G has first been reported by G. Edelman and his associates. The two identical heavy chains (H) are linked in the *hinge region* by sulfhydryl bonds (–S–S–). Each of the light chains (L) is linked by a single sulfhydryl bond to the N-terminal half of an H-chain. The constant region of the H-chains (C_H1, C_H2, C_H3) determines the class to which an immunoglobulin belongs (human IgG is shown in the figure). Light chains may be κ or λ types irrespective of the class of immunoglobulin in which they occur. Amino acid sequence analysis of a large number of κ chains has shown that except for the Inv genetic marker (in position 191) they are identical in the constant (C_L) regions. If we disregard the hypervariable regions (HV) in amino acid positions 24–34, 50–56, and 89–97, the variable portions of human κ chains (V_L) can be subdivided into three subgroups on the basis of amino acid composition. Different κ subgroups are always linked to κ and not to λ type C_L regions. However, each subgroup may be linked to either of the allelic (Inv) forms of the C_L region, suggesting that at least two genes control the synthesis of a single polypeptide. Interestingly, differentiation into subgroups (3 κ and 5 λ subgroups) apparently occurred early in mammalian development, since the difference in amino acid composition of human κ chain subgroups does not exceed the differences among human and mouse basic κ chain sequences. Hypervariable regions of the light chain (HV) are confined to amino acids 24–34, 50–56, and 89–97. The hypervariability determines the contribution of the L-chain to the specificity of the immunoglobulin molecule in its reaction with antigen. Amino acids 23 and 88 are brought into juxtaposition by an intrachain sulfhydryl linkage. Thus, the hypervariable regions (24–34 and 89–97) are brought into approximation, apparently, assuring apposition to a relatively small antigenic determinant.

In IgG the constant region of the heavy (γ) chain can be divided into three portions (C_H1, C_H2, and C_H3) each of which apparently can undergo a specific secondary function (independently of the specificity of the primary antigen-binding function of antibody). Thus, complement appears to be bound at the C_H2 region. C_H2 is also the site of attachment of the carbohydrate that forms part of the constitution of IgG. H-chains are divided into subgroups on the basis of variance of composition of variable region amino acids other than those constituting the hypervariable region. Apparently any subgroup of H-chain may be joined to any of the eight known classes of heavy chains of immunoglobulin (γ_1, γ_2, γ_3, and γ_4 chains in IgG$_1$, IgG$_2$, IgG$_3$, and IgG$_4$ respectively; μ chain in IgM, ϵ chain in IgE, and a_1 and a_2 chains in IgA$_1$ and IgA$_2$). An intrachain sulfhydryl bridge brings H-chain amino acids 22 and 98 into juxtaposition. As a consequece the three hypervariable regions from amino acids 31–37, 86–91, and 101–110 are brought close together, thus apparently assuring their direct contact upon specific reaction with a relatively small antigenic determinant. Recombination studies of L- and H-chains have shown that both chains participate in the specific binding with antigen.

4

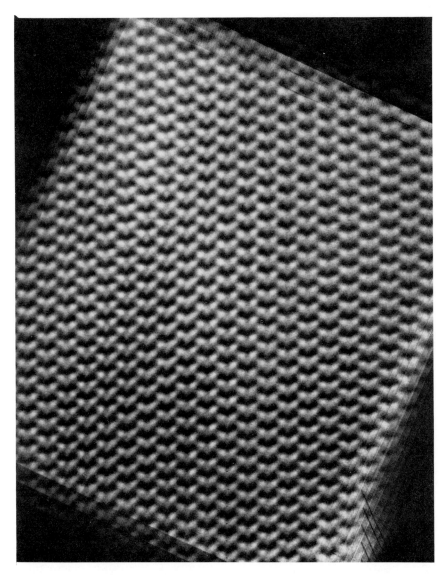

Fig. 1-2 The structure of a myeloma IgG that crystallizes spontaneously on cooling has been studied by X-ray crystallography and negative staining electron microscopy. In order to eliminate random noises of high resolution electron microscopy multiple exposures of the original micrograph were made on printing paper, moving the paper between each exposure in the direction of the crystal periodicity by a distance equal to the periodicity. This procedure was then repeated in different directions of periodicity. From L. W. Labaw and D. R. Davies, *J. Ultrastruct. Res.,* **40**:349, 1972.

the bulk of IgG is excluded from the column (eluting with the starting buffer along with haptoglobulin, an iron-conveying serum protein) although the remainder of serum proteins and other classes of immunoglobulins along with some of the IgG are retained. The molecular weight of IgG is between 145,000 and 156,000. Its specific Y–shape (Fig. 1-1) is suggested by degradation studies and confirmed by electron microscopy (Fig. 1-2). There are four N–terminal amino acids (sometimes with masked amino groups). Therefore, the molecule consists of four chains. Digestion with papain leads to a crystalline fragment Fc and two heterogeneous fragments Fab. If myeloma IgG is digested with papain, both Fab fragments are identical. Therefore, an individual IgG molecule possesses three domains, two identical Fab domains and one Fc domain. Each Fab fragment contains one specific combining site for antigen. Fab blocks the reaction of antigen with native antibody and competitively inhibits the secondary phenomena observed upon reaction of antigen with native antibody. Fab has been used as a specific blocking reagent in immunocytochemistry (page 157). The cleavage into three fragments by papain is due to a preferential attack of the cysteine-activated enzyme on the *hinge region* of IgG. This region possesses unusual flexibility and permits considerable freedom of angular orientation of the Fab domains in relation to each other and to the Fc domain. Because of the identity of both Fab fragments from a single IgG molecule, both specific combining sites are also identical. The freedom of orientation of the Fab fragments permits binding of both antibody sites from a single IgG molecule to two antigenic determinants occurring on a single structure at intervals of varying periodicities [Fig. 6–1 (I)]. Binding with both specific combining sites is important in immunocytochemical reactions as it squares the binding avidity of reaction with a single site and insures, thereby, minimal dissociation of reacted antibody during subsequent processing of tissue.

On mild reduction in the presence of hydrogen bond-breaking agents, such as urea, IgG separates into two identical light (L) chains (about 214 amino acids each) and two identical heavy (H) chains (about 446 amino acids each). Both L- and H-chains have variable N-terminal and constant C-terminal regions. L chains are parts of the Fab fragment only and not of the Fc fragment. Each L chain is bound at its C-terminal or pentultimate amino acid to an H chain with a single sulfhydryl bond. When separated L- and H-chains are acetylated, they will still recombine on admixture. Therefore, urea or propionic acid must be present during the separation of L- and H-chains by gel filtration after reduction. The noncovalent bonding of the L- and H-chains is due to considerable homology of their amino acid sequences. This homology involves the constant as well as variable regions. Thus, when separated L- and H-chains from anti-A and anti-B are allowed to recombine in a single mixture, the L-chains from anti-A will home with a high probability to the H-chains of anti-A and the L-chains from anti-B to the H-chains of anti-B.

The Fc fragment consists of the C-terminal portions of the H-chains, which are constant; hence, the crystalline nature of Fc even if obtained from nonhomogeneous IgG. One sulfhydryl bond in the rabbit, two in man, and three in the guinea pig link both H-chains in the hinge region.

Nisonoff has shown that limited digestion with pepsin fragments the Fc portion of IgG while leaving the Fab portions and the hinge region intact. The resulting $F(ab')_2$ fragment (Fig. 4-1) contains both specific antibody combining sites still bound covalently by sulfhydryl linkage. Fragments containing only one specific combining site (Fab') can be obtained from $F(ab')_2$ by mild reduction even in the absence of hydrogen bond-breaking agents, since both H-chains are held together by only a small sequence of amino acids. Upon reoxidation $F(ab')_2$ is reconstituted. As the linkage is in a constant region of the H-chains, Fab' fragments of different antibody specificities may recombine: the antibodies of dual specificities so obtained have gained much importance in immunocyto-chemistry (Chapter 4).

THE PRIMARY FUNCTION OF ANTIBODIES: SPECIFIC ANTIGEN BINDING

If one prepares an antigen by coupling a *hapten,* such as a small peptide of known amino sequence, with a *carrier,* such as a large protein molecule, immunization, if successful, yields in most instances antibodies reactive with the hapten and antibodies reactive with the carrier. Even the antihaptenic antibodies consist of a heterogeneous group, most of them specific for the terminal amino acid, many for the terminal and the pentultimate amino acid, and a lesser and lesser proportion for an increasingly larger sequence of amino acids. Few antibodies react with a sequence larger than four to seven amino acids away from the terminal amino acid. The larger the number of amino acids with which the antihapten antibody reacts the stronger the binding: the antibody is said to have a high *avidity.* High avidity means close fit with the respective amino acid sequence. Hence, high avidity to an antigen means high specificity and low *cross reactivity* with antigenic determinants of different amino acid sequences. Although with purified antibodies (page 14) not more than four amino acids were found to contribute to binding, the limiting size of an antigenic determinant is probably closer to a sequence of seven amino acids, monosaccharide or nucleotide residues. Purification of antibodies usually selects those with low binding avidities apparently leaving antibodies reactive with more than four amino acids in the nonpurified residue (page 47).

It is not unlikely that the antibodies with high binding avidities that react with a sequence of more than four amino acids constitute only a small, although important fraction of total, measurable antipeptide antibody found in an antiserum.

The reaction of antibody and antigen is reversible. High avidity implies low reversibility. In the development and application of immunocytochemical methods, we must be aware of reversibility because in immunocytochemical staining one usually applies a small volume of antibody-containing reagent and then washes with a large volume of buffer. This causes some dissociation even though with most good antibodies the binding reaction is much faster than the dissociation reaction. Antibodies of good avidity have average intrinsic association constants in the range of 10^5–10^9 per mole, but antibodies of lower avidities are useful in immunocytochemistry when binding with tissue antigens occurs with both antibody specific sites.

In tests for primary binding of antibodies, varying amounts of antigen or hapten are added to constant amounts of antibodies. The ratio of bound to free antigen or hapten is then determined. This ratio can be established by equilibrium dialysis of a radiolabeled hapten against an antibody-containing solution. Alternatively, binding of hapten with purified antibody can be measured directly by fluorescence quenching provided the hapten possesses absorbencies between 300 to 400 nm, as does dinitrophenol: free antibody absorbs light at 280 nm and emits at 350 nm. A dinitrophenol molecule bound in a molecule of antidinitrophenol quenches the fluorescence emission of its Fab portion. Bound radiolabeled haptens or certain antigens can also be evaluated by precipitation of the immunoglobulin in half-saturated ammonium sulfate solution. Hapten or antigen bound with antibody is precipitated, and the amount of free hapten or antigen remaining in solution is measured. The method is restricted to free antigens that are soluble in half-saturated ammonium sulfate solution. Finally, primary binding of antigen with antibody can be determined by the effect of bound antibody on electrophoresis, zonal sedimentation, or gel filtration of the antigen.

THE PRECIPITIN REACTION

Immunoglobulin G possesses two combining sites. Most antigens possess multiple combining sites. Hence, under suitable proportions antigen and antibody form large aggregates that precipitate out of solution. The size of the aggregates does not only depend on the number of combining sites of antigen and antibody but also on binding avidities. If binding avidity is high, aggregates form rapidly, and dissociation of aggregates becomes negligible. However, if an antibody preparation contains a large proportion of antibodies with low binding avidities, polymer formation is slow and not all antigen or antibody in solution may precipitate, irrespective of the proportion of the reactants. Furthermore, immune precipitates obtained with antibodies with low binding avidities may have high solubilities. It follows that estimation of protein contents of an immune precipitate does not necessarily evaluate all the antibody in solution.

Three zones can be distinguished in the precipitin reaction of antigen and antibody: an *antibody excess* zone in which no free antigen remains in solution; an *equivalence* zone in which neither free antigen nor free antibody are detected in solution; and an *antigen excess* zone in which both free antigen as well as soluble antigen-antibody complexes are in solution. Complexes of antibody and excess antigen are soluble because in excess many antigen molecules combine with antibody by only one of their antigenic determinants and, thus, prevent excessive growth of chains of alternating antigen and antibody. Soluble complexes can be obtained in pure form by precipitating antibody with antigen in equivalence and dissolving the precipitate in excess antigen. As this requires the breaking of multiple antigen-antibody bonds, it is a slow reaction that is only partially complete even when large excesses of antigen are used with continuous agitation. Much denaturation of protein ensues. To obtain good yields of antigen-antibody complex with little excess of antigen, as needed in some immunocytochemical applications, more efficient methods of preparation are used (page 132).

Immunodiffusion is a precipitin reaction in semisolid media. As a solution of antigen diffuses against a solution of antibody, a line of precipitation forms at a point of contact where optimal proportions for precipitation have been established (Fig. 2–7). If the antigen solution consists of a variety of components that evoke different antibodies, a number of lines is likely to form as the rate of diffusion of each antigen component is different. A comparison of two or more different antigen preparations against a single antibody solution establishes antigenic identity or diversity depending on whether the antigen preparations form a common line with the antibody preparation (*line of identity*) or whether they form independent lines that cross over at their point of contact (*line of diversity*). *Spur formation* at the point of contact means partial identity: the spur is due to unshared antigenic determinants present in one of the antigens in addition to those shared with the other antigen.

In *immunoelectrophoresis* immunoglobulins are first separated by gel electrophoresis and then analyzed by immunodiffusion either with specific antigen or with immunoglobulin specific against antigenic determinants of the electrophoresed immunoglobulins. The sensitivity of immunoelectrophoresis can be increased by *autoradiography*. After formation of immunodiffusion bands of electrophoresed immunoglobulin with antiimmunoglobulin and removal of soluble components by washing, radiolabeled antigen specific to the electrophoresed immunoglobulin is added, and after additional incubation and washing the preparation is applied to a sensitive photographic emulsion.

IMMUNOGLOBULIN CLASSES AND THE SECONDARY, BIOLOGIC FUNCTION OF ANTIBODIES

The primary binding of antibodies with antigen is responsible for only a few of their biologic functions. Antibodies may bind with the surface of a virus and prevent its cellular attachment and infectivity. Antibodies may cause pernicious anemia by reacting with intrinsic factor and preventing its binding of vitamin B12 (page 226). An antibody may prevent tetanus by combining with tetanus toxin. The reaction of multivalent antigens and antibodies may form large aggregates that affect the course of an immune response. In general, however, the primary reaction of antibody within antigen in itself neither causes the immune elimination of an antigen nor the immune destruction of a cell. These are secondary phenomena that are mediated by properties of the constant regions of the H chains and are specific to the class of antibodies involved.

All classes of immunoglobulins possess a basic 4-chain structure similar to that of IgG. The molecular weights of these 4-chain units differ slightly because of different lengths of H-chains and because of different carbohydrate contents. The L-chains and the variable portions of the H-chains are not class specific. In IgA monomers or dimers of the basic 4-chain structure occur. IgM consists of pentamers of the basic 4-chain structure. The heavy chain of IgM (μ chain) possesses about 500 amino acid residues and contains oligosaccharides attached at 5 sites. The molecular weight of the pentameric IgM molecule is about 1,000,000. Each of the two μ chains in the monomer is joined to an adjacent monomer by a single sulfhydryl bond. The Fc-μ fragment obtained by papain digestion is an annular structure still joined by sulfhydryl bonds that form the central disk of the pentameric molecule. Of the ten specific combining sites of IgM, five are functionally available.

The *complement* system is a series of circulating proteins (proenzymes, enzymes, and substrates) that mediate many of the physiologic effects of antigen-antibody reactions. A sequence of 11 interacting proteins (C1q, C1r, C1s, and C2 to C9) and their activated derivatives is sometimes involved. The activated components three to nine are effector substances directed mainly towards surface properties of cells, causing cell lysis (cytotoxicity) or preparing cells for phagocytosis. Often specific functions of cells are activated, such as a release of histamine from mast cells and platelets, leukotaxis, smooth-muscle contraction, and promotion of blood coagulation.

IgM and IgG activate the complement sequence by the C1,4,2 mechanism. The process is initiated by fixation of C1q, a unique property of IgM and IgG (IgG_3, IgG_1, and IgG_2 subclasses in man). Aggregation of these immunoglobulins enhances their binding qualities for C1q in proportion to the size of the aggregates. Therefore, unaggregated IgM that can be considered a five subunit aggregate is about 15 times as active as non-aggregated IgG. IgM or IgG polymerized by reaction with polyvalent antigens (possessing multiple antigenic determinants) are much more effective than the unreacted antibodies. A single molecule of IgM bound specifically to an antigen-bearing membrane may activate the sequence of events leading eventually to lysis of the membrane. IgG on the other hand must be closely packed on a membrane to initiate binding of C1q firm enough to lead to eventual membrane lysis with a high probability. Therefore, large amounts of IgG are needed for cytotoxicity while small amounts of IgM suffice.

Activation of the complement system proceeds by cleavage of the labile components C1,4,2,3, and 5 that even in solution are fairly unstable in contrast to the typical effector components C6,7,8, and 9 that usually appear electrophoretically homogeneous. The C1 subunit, C1q, reacts with the immune complex that induces C1r to activate C1s to the enzyme $C\overline{1s}$. The enzyme has two natural substrates: C4 and C2. The reaction product is another enzyme ($C\overline{4,2}$) that can be assembled in solution or on a surface at or near the bound antibody. The C4 subunit of this enzyme possesses, however, a site that specifically attaches itself to the immunoglobulin complement receptor region. The resulting cell antibody enzyme complex ($EAC\overline{4,2}$) acts as a *convertase* on C3. Up until this step, the reaction is specific to the immune systems. The mechanism cannot be duplicated by nonimmunologic models. Interestingly the reaction is also highly efficient up until this step: a single molecule of cell bound IgM reacted with a single subunit of C4, and a single subunit of C4 bound to a single subunit of C2 can initiate a reaction that leads to eventual membrane lysis and cell lysis. The subsequently utilized components C3-C9 not only possess biologic activity but, in addition, may be activated by other mechanisms that do not require convertase ($C\overline{4,2}$).

Convertase splits C3 into C3a and C3b. C3a is a small fragment released into solution that possesses the properties of anaphylatoxin and is responsible for the chemotactic activity of leukocytes. C3b, the larger fragment, possesses high affinity for cell membranes. Immunocytochemically it localizes over a much wider zone on a cell membrane than the activators responsible for its release (pages 73 and 158). C3b when attached to cells makes them susceptible to enhanced phagocytosis and to immune adherence. The subsequently reacting components of the complement system attach to the cell-bound C3b. An inactivator cleaves C3b in solution. The inactivator also releases into solution a fragment from the cell bound C3b, but the unreleased fragment still retains biologic activity.

C5 is enzymatically cleaved, and C5,6, and 7 probably attach as a trimolecular complex. C5 causes a morphologic alteration of the cell surface, but lysis only occurs after attachment of C8 and 9.

An *alternate pathway* of complement activation bypasses IgM and IgG and their reaction with antigen and C1,4, and 2. A *proactivator* (properdin) reacts with certain substances such as inulin, zymosan, bacterial endotoxin, or cobra venom to form a cleavage product that activates C3 into C3a and C3b.

Some IgG subclasses display specific *cytophilic* activity for macrophages. The phenomenon may be important in concentrating antigen on the macrophage surface in some pathways of antibody production (page 206).

Transport of immunoglobulin through membranes, such as placental membranes, is an active process almost uniquely characteristic for IgG. IgM is essentially intravascular, but IgG is also found in extravascular fluids.

IgA is the main immunoglobulin of human secretions, such as colostrum, milk, nasal secretions, saliva, and gastrointestinal secretions. Two subclasses are determined by an α_1 and α_2 chain. In most cases the α_2 chains are bound to the L-chains without a disulfide linkage. Alpha chains and IgA possess a tendency towards spontaneous polymerization. Most of the circulating IgA, however, is monomeric (basic 4-chain structure). The bulk of the secreted IgA is dimeric. The dimeric form is associated with a *secretory component,* a carbohydrate-containing β globulin. Some of the secretory component is also free in secretions. The secretory component confers upon IgA an increased resistance against proteolytic enzymes, such as found in secretions. The *junction* (J) *chain* is an additional peptide found in polymeric but not in monomeric IgA. B. Bloth and S.-E Svehag have shown by electron microscopy that dimeric IgA has great flexibility about the point where both Fc regions are joined. The IgA found in secretions is produced locally as monomers by the lymphoid cell aggregates usually present in large quantities in submucosal areas and beneath the epithelial surface of exocrine glands. Dimerization is a function of the epithelium.

IgE, discovered by K. and T. Ishizaka, is found in very small quantities in human and animal sera and carries the unique property of sensitizing *species homologous* tissue towards allergic reactions (reaginic antibody in man, homocytotropic antibody in animals). IgE myeloma protein is a carbohydrate-containing 4-chain immunoglobulin with a molecular weight of about 190,000. IgE binds specifically with the surface of basophils in circulation and mast cells in tissues, and acts as receptor for specific antigens. Upon reaction with such antigen, the cells degranulate; histamine and other substances are released, and the typical effects of reaginic hypersensitivity ensue. The binding to these cells can be studied by radioautography if degranulation and histamine release are prevented by ethylene diamine tetra-acetate, thus, permitting cellular identification. Using radioiodinated anti-ϵ with preparations of human cells or tissues and developing the reaction with a sensitive photographic emulsion, silver grains are found only on basophils and mast cells, thus, identifying these cells as the only cells that have bound IgE from the serum of their donor.

When serum from a ragweed-sensitive patient is added to normal leukocytes, exposure to ragweed allergen releases histamine from the basophils in the preparation. If myeloma IgE is added to normal leukocytes, exposure to anti-IgE also releases histamine. This shows that it is the IgE moiety in both reactions that is responsible for the specific attachment at basophils and the release of histamine. IgE may be a predisposing factor in immune complex disease (page 223).

Conceivably the binding of IgE to cells may be responsible for the finding of only low residual levels of this immunoglobulin in circulation. There may exist other immunoglobulins that are even more strongly bound than IgE and are, therefore, never found in circulation. This may be the case in delayed sensitivity, a specific immunologic phenomenon mediated by cells and not by immunoglobulin in circulation.

IDIOTYPIC ANTIBODIES

When we immunize mice of one strain with an immunoglobulin of another strain, we obtain antibodies against *allotypic* determinants. However, if we immunize mice with immunoglobulin obtained from the same strain, we usually do not obtain antibodies because animals are normally immune tolerant of their own antigenic determinants (pages 208 and 215). A homogeneous immunoglobulin, such as BALB/c myeloma IgA S63, possesses a unique sequence in its hypervariable region. Normal BALB/c mice at best contain only a trace of this particular hypervariable sequence among all their heterogeneous immunoglobulins. The amount of this sequence may well be below the threshold for induction of immune tolerance. Thus when normal BALB/c mice are immunized with protein S63, tolerance is broken and antibodies form. These antibodies are specific to the hypervariable region of protein S63. Antibodies to hypervariable regions of immunoglobulin have been called *idiotypic* by A. Nisonoff.

IgA S63 possesses antibody specificity for phosphoryl choline. If antisera are produced by this protein in an allogenic strain of mice, idiotypic antibodies can be identified after absorption with insolubilized protein S129, a myeloma IgA from BALB/c mice with antidinitrophenol reactivity.

Idiotypic antibodies can also be produced in heterologous species. Protein 315 is a mouse myeloma IgA with anti-2,4-dinitrophenol activity. To obtain idiotypic antibodies from rabbits immunized with protein 315, the antiserum is first absorbed with a mouse myeloma IgA of different specificity. The antiserum is reabsorbed with protein 315 that has been reacted with N-bromacetyl-N'-2,4-dinitrophenylethylenediamine. This compound is an *affinity label* that reacts immunospecifically with the combining sites of protein 315 and covalently with lysine groups in or near the combining sites. Absorption of the rabbit antiserum with the affinity-labeled protein 315 removes, therefore, antibodies to all its antigenic determinants except some of those that are in or near the specific combining sites. The absorbed antiserum becomes idiotypic. The reaction of idiotypic antibody with protein 315 is inhibited by 2,4-dinitrophenol and analogous ligands indicating that the idiotypic antibody is, indeed, specific for the specific combining site of protein 315.

A. Sher, E. Lord, and M. Cohn have shown that protein 107 (a BALB/c mouse myeloma IgA antiphosphoryl choline) reacts with the idiotypic antibody produced with protein S63. In this case, however, the reaction is not altered by the presence of phosphoryl choline. Conceivably the antibodies are not truly idiotypic but specific to a rare subgroup of IgA that is expressed in tumors S63 and 107 and is not abundant in normal BALB/c mice.

M. Kuettner, A. Wong, and A. Nisonoff found that idiotypic antibodies reactive with a specific mouse antihaptenic myeloma globulin cross react to a *lesser extent* with myeloma globulin specific to the same hapten from mice of different strains. The results indicate that idiotypic specificity may provide genetic markers for the variable regions of immunoglobulin polypeptide chains.

Idiotypic antibodies are one of the possible causative mechanisms for autoimmune disease (page 217).

PURIFICATION OF ANTIBODIES

Antibodies can be purified from serum by precipitation with specific antigen. The washed precipitate is dissociated at low pH and antigen separated from antibody at this pH by gradient sedimentation. Alternatively, the precipitate can be dissociated by certain salts, such as magnesium chloride or potassium thiocyanate. At 2.5 M concentration, solution of immune precipitates is only partial, while at higher concentrations denaturation of antibody is extensive. Salt-dissociated antibody and antigens can be separated by gel filtration columns equilibriated with the dissociating ions. Antibodies to haptenic determinants, such as 2,4-dinitrophenol (DNP), can be purified by (1) precipitation with DNP-conjugated ovalbumin, (2) dissociation of the precipitate with DNP-lysine, (3) separation of antigen (DNP-ovalbumin) from antibody by gel filtration in the presence of DNP-lysine, and (4) removal of DNP-lysine by dialysis, first against buffered DNP, and finally against buffered saline. The DNP-lysine-antibody complex is soluble because of the monovalence (single combining site) of the DNP haptenic group.

Immunoabsorption may be employed instead of immune precipitation. An *immunoabsorbent* is an insolubilized antigen. Antigen may be insolubilized by polymerization, as for instance with glutaraldehyde, or by reaction with derivatized cellulose, or other insoluble matrices, such as bromacetyl-cellulose, or by entrapment in cross-linked microporous polyacrylamide gel. Elution is carried out under conditions resembling those of dissociation of immune precipitates. Immunoabsorbents have the advantage that only antibody and not antigen is eluted, thus, bypassing the need of lengthy separation procedures. However, immunoabsorbents require more antigen than immune precipitates.

In general, specific purification recovers only part of the antibodies removed from serum. The better the avidity of antibody the poorer the yield. The antibodies of highest binding avidities, which often comprise only a small fraction of total antibody, are usually not dissociated from immune precipitates or immunoabsorbents.

The yields in protein, but not in average binding avidity, are usually higher with immunoabsorbents than with immune precipitates. In immunoabsorption both low and high avidity antibodies are bound, and low avidity antibodies are recovered in high yield. In immune precipitation the antibodies with low avidities usually remain in solution. The selection of higher avidity antibodies in the immune precipitate diminishes recovery in terms of antibody protein, although, the average binding avidity of the recovered antibody is probably higher than with immunoabsorbents.

Immune precipitates selecting for antibodies with high avidity can be obtained by precipitation in antibody excess: high avidity antibodies bind antigen rapidly and leave a large proportion of low avidity antibodies in solution. For this reason T. Ternyck and S. Avrameas obtained especially low yields of antibodies purified from immune precipitates prepared in antibody excess. The question of high avidity of purified antibodies is important in several immunocytochemical methods (Chapters 4 and 6).

REFERENCES

Augener, W., Grey, H. M., Cooper, N. R., and Müller–Eberhard, H. J. The reaction of monomeric and aggregated immunoglobulins with C1. *Immunochemistry*, 8:1011, 1971.

Bloth, B. and Svehag, S.-E. Further studies on the ultrastructure of dimeric IgA of human origin. *J. Exp. Med.*, 133:1035, 1971.

Brient, B. W., Haimerich, J., and Nisonoff, A. Reaction of anti-idiotypic antibody with the hapten binding site of a myeloma protein. *Proc. Nat. Acad. Sci.*, U.S., 68:3136, 1971.

Capra, J. P., Winchester, R. W., and Kunkel, H. G. Hypergammaglobulinemic purpura. Studies on the unusual anti-γ-globulins characteristic of the sera of these patients. *Medicine*, 50:125, 1971.

Carrel, S. and Barandun, S. Protein-containing polyacrylamide gels: Their use as immunoabsorbents of high capacity. *Immunochemistry*, 8:39, 1971.

Edelman, G. M., Cunningham, B. A., Gall, W. E., Gottlieb, P. D., Rutisha, U., and Waxdal, M. J. The covalent structure of an entire γG immunoglobulin molecule. *Proc. Nat. Acad. Sci.*, U.S., 63:78, 1969.

Hood, L. E. Two genes, one polypeptide—fact or fiction?" *Fed. Proc.*, 31:177, 1972.

Ishizaka, K., Tomioko, H., and Ishizaka, T. Mechanisms of passive sensitization. I. Presence of IgE and IgG molecules on human leukocytes. *J. Immunol.*, 105:1459, 1970.

Kehoe, J. M. and Capra, J. D. Localization of two additional hypervariable regions in immunoglobulin heavy chains. *Proc. Nat. Acad. Sci.*, U.S., 68:2019, 1971.

Kuettner, M. G., Wang, A. L., and Nisonoff, A. Quantitative investigations of idiotypic antibodies. II. Idiotypic specificity as a potential marker for the variable region of mouse immunoglobulin polypeptide chains. *J. Exp. Med.*, 135:579, 1972.

Labaw, L. W. and Davies, D. R. The molecular outline of human γ G1 immunoglobulin from an EM study of crystals. *J. Ultrastruct. Res.*, 40:349, 1972.

MacKenzie, M. R., Creevy, N., and Heh, M. The interaction of human IgM and C1q. *J. Immunol.*, 106:65, 1971.

Mayer, M. M. Highlights of complement research during the past twenty-five years. *Immunochemistry*, 7:485, 1970.

Mayer, M. M., Miller, J. A., and Shin, H. S. A specific method for purification of the second component of guinea pig complement and a chemical evaluation of the one-hit theory. *J. Immunol.*, 105:237, 1970.

Putnam, F. W., Shinizu, A., Paul, C., and Shinoda, T. Variation and homology in immunoglobulin heavy chains. *Fed. Proc.,* **31**:193, 1972.

Ruddy, S., Hunsicker, L. G., and Austen, K. F. C3b inactivator of man. III. Further purification and production of antibody to C3bINA. *J. Immunol.,* **108**:657, 1972.

Sarma, V. R., Davis, D. R., Labaw, L. W., Silverton, E. W., and Terry, W. D. Crystal structure of an immunoglobulin molecule by X-ray diffraction and electron microscopy. *Cold Spring Harbor Symposia Quant. Biol.,* **36**:413, 1971.

Sher, A., Lord, E., and Cohn, M. Reconstitution from subunits of the hapten binding sites and idiotypic determinants of mouse antiphosphorylcholine myeloma proteins. *J. Immunol.,* **107**:1226, 1971.

Ternynck, T. and Avrameas, S. Effects of electrolytes and distilled water on antigen-antibody complexes. *Biochem. J.,* **125**:297, 1971.

Chapter 2

Immunofluorescence

In the early forties immunology had established itself as a science. The word immunochemistry had been coined; quantitation of immunologic techniques had become the requirement of the day, and Kabat and Mayer were writing their first edition of *Experimental Immunochemistry*. Massugi had produced experimental glomerulonephritis by injection into rats of duck anti-rat kidney serum, and Kay had shown that the lesion was produced by an autoimmune mechanism. Rheumatic fever was an enigma, and the question was timely whether its characteristic lesion, the Aschoff nodule, contained a specific antigen, perhaps a streptococcal product, or whether it was an expression of autoimmune hypersensitivity, or both. These were the days when two pages in the *Proceedings of the Society of Experimental Biology and Medicine* and eleven pages in the *Journal of Immunology* brought the first communication on the labeling of antibodies with fluorescent groups and the detection by fluorescent miscroscopy of pneumococcal antigens in sections of pneumococcus-infected tissue.

When these first reports of Coons appeared, immunology was already contributing a large proportion of articles in the *Journal of Experimental Medicine*. Yet, little was on the horizon to anticipate the far-reaching role that immunology would play in areas of biology and medicine beyond immunity and allergy. For as long as ten years, Coons' first communication found no followers. Use of fluorescein-conjugated antibodies was considered a difficult technique. Indeed, the technique did not become easier when nonspecific staining had been discovered by Coons in the early fifties in a report that also gave more details about preparation of fluorescein isocyanate, conjugation with antibodies, and preparation of microtome sections for staining with fluorescein-conjugated antibodies. The necessity of low ratios of fluorescein to protein had become apparent, and the removal of nonspecific staining by absorption with liver powder has become an empirical practice. What is more important, however, by then science had progressed to a point that the genius of Albert Coons found appropriate recognition. It must have been Coons' conviction in the ultimate importance of his work that made him persist in following his original discovery with further work ten years later, thereby, initiating immuno-cytochemistry as that subdiscipline of immunology that was primarily responsible for bringing pathology into immunology and for bringing from the category of unknown to that of defined etiology a greater number of diseases than any other advance in medical sciences. As a result, today 45% of articles in a general medical journal, such as the *Lancet,* rely on immunology as compared to 5% in the pre-immunofluorescence days.

In the ensuing years immunofluorescence rapidly established itself as the first application of immunology that addressed itself beyond such purely immunologic inquiries, as nature of antibodies and mechanisms of immunity and hypersensitivity. By being able, in principle, to detect any antigenic and insoluble tissue constituent *in situ* immunofluorescence became the most versatile and specific tool of cytochemistry capable of correlating quantitative chemical information with anatomic structure. These new applications go beyond the scope of immunology proper and permit the coining of the word "immunocytochemistry."

When tissues are stained with routine, nonspecific stains for histology and pathology, such as eosin and hematoxylin, the color contrast is sufficient that bright red and deep blue can easily be seen in the light microscope despite the thinness of a 2–6 μ section. Offhand it appears conceivable, therefore, to dye antibodies in solution and use in turn the colored antibody for specific localization of tissue antigen in microscopy. Indeed, antibodies can react with dyes just as well as tissue constituents do. Azo-dyes give some of the strongest colors. They react with the tyrosine groups in the protein molecule. The reaction of antibody with azo-dye must be restricted to less than ten molucules of dye per molecule of antibody because increasing extent of reaction progressively destroys antibody activity and, in many cases, also interferes with antibody solubility. When only a small number of dye molecules has reacted with antibody and antibody activity has been largely retained, the resulting solution of antibody immunoglobulin is nonetheless deeply colored at the high immunoglobulin concentration viewed in a test tube. However, the color is insufficient to be recognized through the microscope in the 1–6 μ thick section necessary for examination of tissue, even if an abundant antigen, such as a viral inclusion body, has reacted with specific antibody. The microscopist would have to distinguish unstained tissue that has full transmission, say 100%, from weakly stained tissue whose transmission is impaired by, say 3%. The difference between 100% and 97% transmission cannot be discerned by the naked eye. Were one to make antibody fluorescent by conjugation of an antibody molecule with one fluorescent group, choosing a strongly absorbing molecule, such as fluorescein isocyanate, a conjugated antibody solution is obtained that absorbs much less light energy than the antibody labeled with ten azo-dye molecules. However, the fluorescent antibody confers bright green fluorescence to specific antigen in tissue sections. (See the color of the book jacket.) The brightness is due to the method of observation. In fluorescence microscopy the light absorbed is of shorter wavelength than the light emitted. Since the light from the light source is partially beyond the visible range and since filters are employed to eliminate the light originating from the light source, the microscopic field is dark except for the specifically stained fluorescent component. Even though the fluorescent tissue component may emit only 1% as much light as is seen in light microscopy under full transmission, this 1% is viewed in a surrounding field having practically zero percent transmission and can, therefore, easily be discerned by the naked eye. In light microscopy when detectability of a colored component is limited by a small difference between two high light intensities, increasing the total light intensity will yield little gain in proportional visibility. In fluorescence microscopy, on the other hand, increase of intensity of the light source does increase the sensitivity because it increases fluorescent emission against a background that still remains dark. Hence, strong light sources and good optics are essential in fluorescence microscopy.

Every organic substance absorbs light at least in the far ultraviolet and dissipates the absorbed energy either in the form of a chemical reaction, or as heat, or as visible light. We may decide, therefore, that a molecule suitable for immunofluorescence will have to possess at least two properties: (1) it must be efficient in absorbing light, (2) it must dissipate the absorbed light largely in the form of emitted light rather than as rotational and vibrational energy. We may want to add that the fluorescent molecule chosen should not be able to absorb at the wavelength at which it emits light, i.e., the fluorescence produced should not be internally quenched. Aliphatic, saturated compounds are not fluorescent. Their electrons are firmly bound and, hence, they absorb light only over a narrow spectral range in the far ultraviolet. Most bonds in these molecules are freely rotating and, hence, their absorbed energy is rapidly dissipated as rotational energy.

Absorbence of light is aided by the addition of loosely bound electrons, especially when they are dissipated over the entire molecule as resonance electrons. One condition leading to this situation is the presence of conjugated double bonds. A second condition is the presence of polar substituents that give the molecule electron donating and electron accepting centers. An example is a quinoline compound with a substituted pyridinium group. Of further aid is resonance dissipation of ions, such as in pseudocyanine (Fig. 2-1) or of electrons if there exist several equivalents of electron distribution (hybridization).

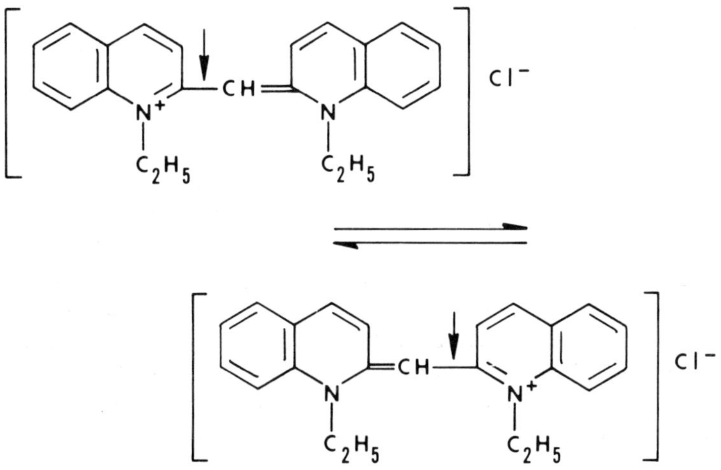

Fig. 2-1 Pseudocyanine. This molecule absorbs light over a wide range of wavelengths. It possesses loosely bound electrons dissipated over the molecule through the conjugated double-bond system and through hybridization effected by the two equivalent ion distribution states shown. The compound is a yellow-red dye. The molecule can rotate in the position of the arrows. Absorbed energy is thus dissipated. Hence, the compound is *not* fluorescent.

In order for a molecule to *emit* its absorbed light as fluorescence, that part of the molecule that is responsible for light absorption must possess a structural rigidity sufficient to prevent dissipation of the energy by rotation. These conditions are fulfilled by the structures of fluorescein and of rhodamine (Fig. 2-2). Another reason for the choice of these markers in immunofluorescence is their greenish and reddish color of emission, respectively, that makes them distinguishable from the bluish autofluorescence of nucleic acids, and protein tryptophane and tyrosine in tissues. The two markers can also be easily distinguished from one another. This permits the simultaneous demonstration of two antigens in the same tissue section by means of two appropriate antibodies, one coupled to fluorescein and the other to rhodamine.

Fluorescein, and rhodamine, and other fluorochromes must be converted to molecules capable of reacting with antibodies under conditions that do not abolish specific antibody activity: the minimal conditions are reaction in aqueous solution at or below room temperature.

To obtain a fluorescein derivative that can be conjugated into protein, nitrofluorescein is synthesized, starting from resorcinol and 4-nitrophthalein anhydride. *Via* nitrophenolphthalein as an intermediate, abstraction of one molecule of water and ring closure yields nitrofluorescein (Fig. 2-3). Two isomers are obtained depending upon which of the two carboxy

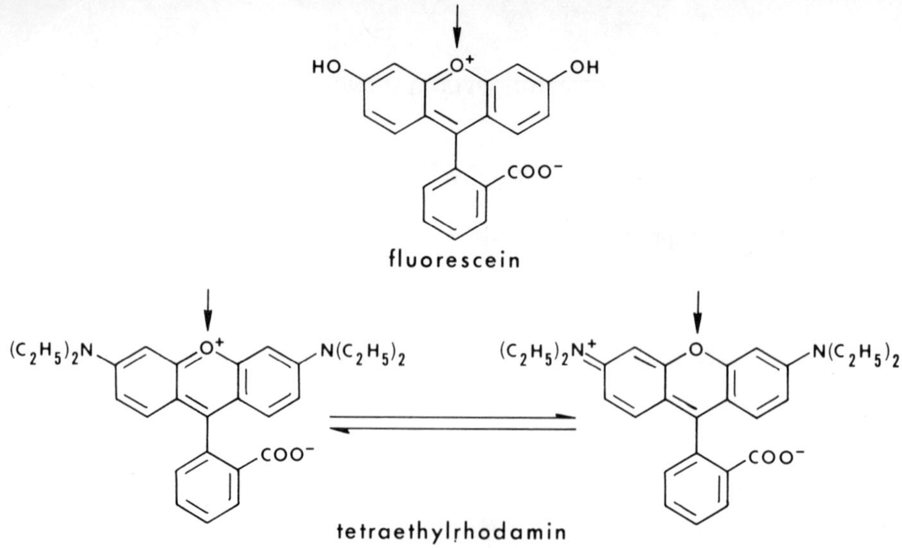

fluorescein

tetraethylrhodamin

Fig. 2-2 Fluorescein and its bis-dialkylamino derivatives absorb light efficiently because of the distribution of π-electrons over the resonating system of three conjugated rings, because of the polarity contributed by the positive and negative charges in the molecule, and because of the dispersion of electrons (loose bonds) contributed by ionic hybridization (two of the resonating forms of rhodamine are shown). The molecules are fluorescent because the light absorbing part of their structures possesses planar rigidity effected in their synthesis by the ring closure at the positions of the arrows.

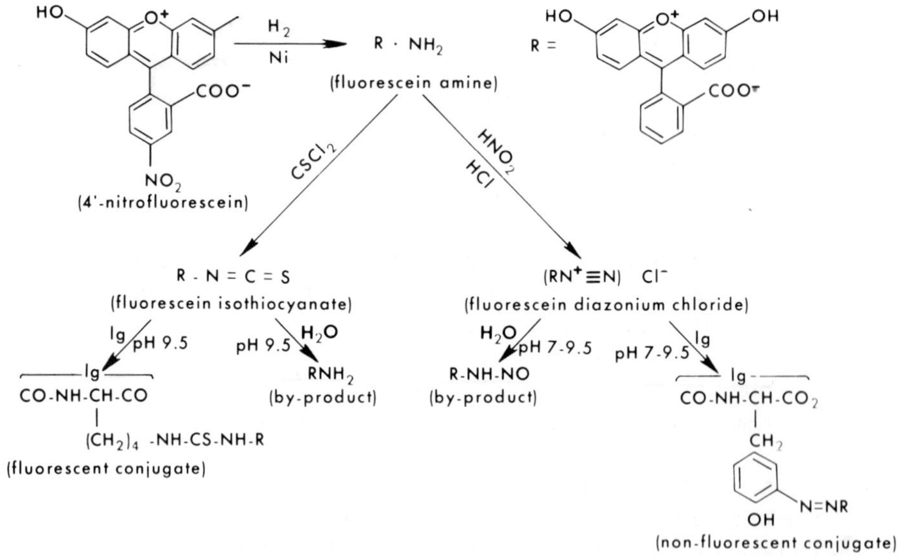

Fig. 2-3 Nitrofluorescein is reduced to the amino compound. To conjugate fluorescein with protein, the isothiocyanate reaction is chosen. Conjugation occurs with the free amino groups of immunoglobulin in aqueous solution (the amino groups of lysine, as shown, or terminal amines on each L- and H-chain). Side reactions with the solvent lead to hydrolysis of the fluorescein isothiocyanate.

Diazotization of the amine would lead to the diazonium salt that can be coupled into tyrosine of immunoglobulin. This reaction is not useful for immunofluorescence with fluorescein because the azo-dye quenches the fluorescence. A side reaction during coupling at slightly alkaline pH is formation of nitrozamine from the diazonium compound.

groups of nitrophthalein condenses with two resorcinol molecules. The isomers are separated, and one of them is reduced to fluorescein amine.

Amines, especially aromatic amines, are convenient starting materials for the preparation of highly reactive derivatives that conjugate with proteins in the cold and in pH ranges (5–9.5) at which denaturation of proteins is minimized. These derivatives include isocyanates and the more soluble isothiocyanates, diazonium salts, and azides. Alternatively, the amines can be reacted directly with protein via carbodiimide.

For use in immunofluorescence, fluorescein amine (or tetramethylrhodamine amine) is condensed with thiophosgene to form the isothiocyanate. Isothiocyanates react with amines (such as primary amino groups in protein) to form thiourea derivatives and with water at alkaline pH to reconstitute the amine from which the isothiocyanate was made. For efficient coupling of fluorescein isothiocyanate with antibody-amine, the pH should not be lower than 9.5. Some of the fluorescein isothiocyanate will be lost because of reaction with water. The resulting fluorescein amine is one of the products that must be separated from the fluorescein-conjugated antibody after conjugation.

Diazonium compounds have been used extensively for labeling of proteins since coupling proceeds rapidly and efficiently in the cold. The reaction leads to formation of azotyrosine and azohistidine bonds. The compounds are usually deep red in color; that is, they absorb blue and green light. It is for this reason that the azo-linkage is not suitable for conjugation of fluorescein with antibody: the greenish fluorescence of fluorescein is quenched by the azo-coupling. However, rhodamine analogues of fluorescein yield fluorescent conjugates via azo-linkage, because the fluorescence emission is in the orange red range and is only partially quenched by the azo-bond. However, the fluorescence is weaker than that obtained with rhodamine isothiocyanate conjugation.

For the preparation of orange-red fluorescein conjugates, rhodamine disulphonic acid is the preferred starting material (Fig. 2-4). The sulfonyl chloride (prepared by reaction with phosphorus pentachloride) reacts with amino groups in the protein.

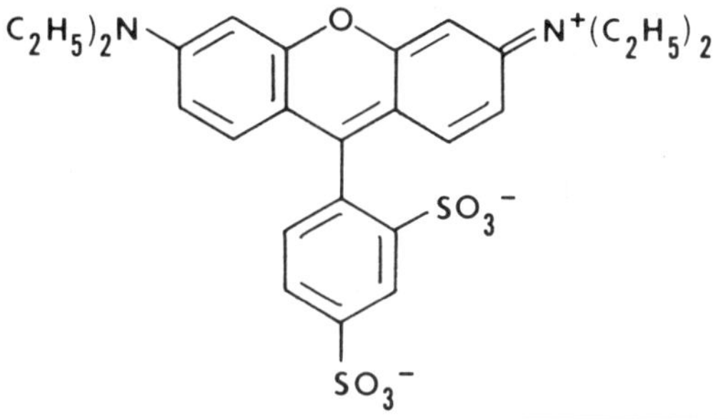

Fig. 2-4 Rhodamine disulfonic acid (Lissamine rhodamine B200).

CONJUGATION OF ANTIBODY WITH
FLUORESCEIN ISOTHIOCYANATE

When reagents containing fluorescein-conjugated antibodies are used for staining of specific antigen in tissue, ideally only the specific antibody should react while the remaining constituents of the reagent are removed by washing. Fortunately, the bulk of the nonspecific constituents of the conjugate are, indeed, so, removed. Therefore, it is not necessary to use purified antibodies (page 14) for reaction with fluorescein isothiocyanate. An immunoglobulin fraction containing specific antibody is quite satisfactory.

Electron hybridization makes strong fluorochromes highly polar substances. In fluorescein two readily ionizable, aromatic hydroxyl groups and one carboxyl group contributed to polarity. Polar groups in an otherwise hydrophobic molecule further nonspecific attachment to tissue constituents, i.e., "staining nonspecificity" (page 46). Furthermore, reaction of isothiocyanate with amino groups of proteins increases the negative charge of the conjugate and, thus, invites nonspecific staining, especially with positively charged proteins such as lysozyme and histones. For these reasons two precautions are essential in the preparation of satisfactory conjugates: removal of all nonconjugated fluorescein (isothiocyanate hydrolysis products, Fig. 2-3) and avoidance of immunoglobulin conjugated with an excessive amount of fluorescein. In serum proteins several amino groups are readily available for reaction with isothiocyanate, but others are buried and less available for reaction. The heterogeneity of immunoglobulins precludes more than an approximate degree of prediction of the extent of conjugation. In any single preparation a wide spectrum in extent of conjugation is obtained requiring separation of the more extensively and less extensively reacted portions of conjugate.

Serum albumin reacts with isothiocyanate faster than immunoglobulin. Consequently, it is not possible to even approximately predict the fluorescein-antibody ratio when isothiocyanate is added to unfractionated antisera. It is essential, therefore, to obtain at least a crude globulin fraction from serum by ammonium or sodium sulfate precipitation. For careful work the immunoglobulin class under study should be isolated chromatographically. The isolation of IgG, at least IgG_2, from crude serum globulin, is a simple procedure (page 27). Goldstein has shown that nonspecific binding of fluorescein isothiocyanate (FITC)-conjugated immunoglobulin with tissue is minimized without greatly affecting the brightness of staining if the molar ratio of FITC to protein (expressed as IgG, molecular weight 150,000) is limited to 1:1 or 2:1. Since in the conjugation of protein with FITC most of the FITC is hydrolyzed, only a portion of the FITC actually couples with the protein. This is another reason why the extent of coupling can be predicted only approximately. Crystalline FITC (available commercially) should be used for a reasonably predictable reaction, or at least a reaction in which the fraction of conjugate possessing 1–2 fluorescein groups per 150,000 molecular weight unit comprises a high proportion of total conjugate. To this end one uses 15–25 μg FITC per mg of IgG or 6–8 moles of FITC per mole of immunoglobulin. Following conjugation two separations are indicated, one of which is essential and the other desirable. Essential is the separation from the conjugate of unconjugated fluorescein (consisting of hydrolysis products, which bind nonspecifically, and conceivably even unreacted FITC that could react covalently with tissue, especially when conjugation is carried out in the cold and staining at room temperature). The separation is best carried out by passage through a column of Sephadex G25.

When most molecules of IgG contain either one or two molecules of fluorescein, Gaussian distribution requires that many molecules of IgG contain no fluorescein. That fraction of total conjugate that possesses fluorescein/protein (Fl/P) ratios in excess of two will increase nonspecific staining. FITC-IgG conjugates of varying Fl/P ratios can be separated on DEAE cellulose. At low ionic strength, near neutrality, unreacted IgG does not bind to the column. Conjugated protein, because of conversion of amino groups to carbamido groups and because of the charge on fluorescein is more negatively charged than unconjugated IgG. Consequently, it becomes bound on the DEAE cellulose column. Binding affinity increases with extent of conjugation. Hence, when the ionic strength of the starting buffer is increased the unconjugated IgG will be followed, in turn with weakly conjugated (Fl/P mole ratio of 1–2) and strongly conjugated protein.

It is necessary to monitor the effluent of the column for fluorescein and protein contents in order to identify the fractions with Fl/P ratios of 1–2. Protein concentration is monitored by absorbence at 280 nm and fluorescein concentration at 495 nm. Fluorescein diacetate is conveniently used as a standard for estimation of conjugated FITC.

For careful work it is of some importance that the determination of the Fl/P ratio is accurate. Unfortunately, the absorption coefficient of fluorescein diacetate at 495 nm is not exactly equal to that of FITC when conjugated with protein. Using ^{14}C-FITC Brighton and Johnson found that in general the optical density (OD) of fluorescein decreases upon conjugation with protein. There is a wide variation among different proteins, and because of the heterogeneity of immunoglobulins it is impossible to derive a generally applicable correction factor.

All these considerations are necessary to obtain optimal conjugates that result in bright fluorescent staining and are encountered with a minimum of nonspecificity. Let us not forget, however, that much if not most of the knowledge gathered by immunofluorescence has been obtained with less than optimal conjugates. Hence, in the following we will detail two procedures for preparation of conjugate, a relatively simple one for detection of abundant antigens of proven characteristics and a more exacting one essential for detection of antigens not necessarily known by other methods to exist within the tissue examined.

Preparation of Fluorescein Isothiocyanate-Immunoglobulin Conjugates (FITC-Ig): Minimal Procedure

Working at 1–6°, dilute the antiserum with an equal volume of water, add an ammonium sulfate solution, saturated in the cold, dropwise and under stirring until 50% saturation is reached. Continue stirring for 20 minutes. Avoid foaming. Centrifuge at 17,500 rpm (Sorvall rotor SS-34) for 15 minutes. Dissolve precipitate in a small volume of water. Reprecipitate by slow addition of ammonium sulfate to 47% saturation. Continue stirring for another 20 minutes and recentrifuge. Dissolve precipitate in a minimum volume of water and dialyze against three changes of 15 liter each of phosphate-buffered saline (PBS). Centrifuge at 17,500 rpm for 10 minutes. Estimate protein concentration of supernate by diluting a small volume with PBS and recording absorbence at 280 nm (protein concentration in mg/ml = OD · 0.62 · dilution factor). If the protein concentration is above 25 mg/ml, calculate the volume that would contain 20 mg/ml. Add $\frac{1}{5}$ of that volume in 0.5 M carbonate bicarbonate buffer, pH 9.5. Then dilute to the calculated volume with PBS (so that the final solution will be 20 mg/ml in protein, 0.1 M in carbonate buffer). Under gentle stirring add 500 μg of crystalline FITC per ml of protein solution. If the original protein concentration is less than 25 mg/ml, add ¼ of its volume in 0.5 M sodium carbonate buffer followed by 25 μg of FITC for each mg of protein. Continue stirring for 24 hours. Remove any precipitate formed in the crude conjugate by centrifugation at 17,500 rpm for 10 minutes.

Suspend Sephadex G25 and decant several times in deaerated PBS at room temperature. Pour a column and reequilibrate at 1–6° by passage of deaerated PBS. Place the crude conjugate onto the column and elute with PBS. Two fluorochrome-containing bands separate visibly. The leading band consists of fluorescein-protein conjugate and of unconjugated protein and is obtained in the void volume. Collect this material. The trailing band contains unreacted fluorescent material (as well as the carbonate buffer). Discard it. Concentrate the collected conjugate by pressure dialysis (preferably on a filter membrane under magnetic stirring). If sterilized by a passage through a Millipore filter, the conjugate is stable for at least a year at 1–6° under protection from light.

The column can be kept indefinitely if slowly, but continually flushed with a deaerated solution of 0.01% sodium azide and equilibriated prior to reuse with PBS devoid of sodium azide.

PREPARATION OF FLUORESCEIN ISOTHIOCYANATE-IMMUNOGLOBULIN G CONJUGATE (FITC-IgG): EXACTING PROCEDURE

The more exacting procedure depends on the ease of separation of IgG (or more precisely, IgG_2) from other immunoglobulins on a diethyl-aminoethyl cellulose column.

Except when noted otherwise the procedure is carried out between 0 and 5°. Antiserum is diluted with an equal volume of saline, and saturated ammonium sulfate solution is added dropwise under agitation to 37% saturation. Stirring is continued for 20 minutes, and the suspension is centrifuged at 14,000 rpm for 15 minutes (Sorvall Rotor SS-34). The precipitate is redissolved in the smallest possible volume of water and dialyzed against three changes of 15 liter each of 0.01 M phosphate buffer, pH 7.5 (*not* PBS). It is of advantage to record the osmolarity or conductivity of the buffer. Completeness of dialysis may be ascertained by assuring that the osmolarity or conductivity of the last dialysis resembles that of the original buffer or by absence of ammonium ion as determined with the Nessler reagent.

For isolation of IgG (which usually comprises the bulk of antibodies in high titered sera) as well as for purification of the conjugate, about 2 gm of DEAE-cellulose (minimum capacity: 0.14 milliequivalents per gm) are used for each ml of dialyzed protein. The DEAE-cellulose is treated with 0.5 N sodium hydroxide solution at room temperature. When the bulk of the cellulose has settled the supernatent suspension, containing some "fines," is decanted and the sediment resuspended in water. Decantation and resuspension in water are continued until the pH of the supernate is approximately 9.0. The sediment is then resuspended in 0.1 M phosphate buffer, pH 7.5, until the pH of the supernate is 7.5. Again the sediment is washed in water until osmolarity or conductivity of the supernate is less than that of the 0.01 M phosphate buffer, pH 7.5. The sediment is then resuspended in the 0.01 M phosphate buffer, pH 7.5, and the suspension, as well as the remainder of the buffer to be washed, are deaerated at 1–5° overnight. Continuing work at 0–5° a column is poured through a wide funnel with approximately ½ of the suspension, taking care to stir the suspension in the funnel in order to avoid banding. The column is then equilibriated with 0.01 M phosphate buffer, pH 7.5, and osmolarity and conductivity of the effluent buffer are again checked. The dialyzed protein, cleared by centrifugation at 35,000 rpm for 10 minutes, is applied to the column and elution is carried out with 0.01 M phosphate buffer, pH 7.5. The absorbence of the effluent is monitored at 280 nm and the eluate fractions with OD's above 0.1 are pooled. An amount of 1.5 M sodium chloride solution is added to bring the sodium chloride concentration to 0.15 M and the material is concentrated by pressure dialysis (preferably with stirring on a membrane such as provided by Amicon ultrafilters). Protein concentration is measured by absorbence at 280 nm and adjusted to 2% in protein, 0.05 M in carbonate and approximately 0.15 N in sodium chloride by dilution with 0.5 M carbonate buffer, pH 9.5, (1⁄10th of the final volume) and 0.15 N sodium chloride solution. Under agitation 15–20 μg of dry crystalline FITC are added per mg of IgG, and the pH is kept at 9.5 with 0.05 M sodium carbonate solution using a pH-stat or manual technique. After one hour the mixture is centrifuged at 17,500 rpm for 10 minutes, and the reaction is terminated by buffer exchange and removal of unreacted FITC. This as well as selection of optimally conjugated IgG is conveniently accomplished by a Sephadex G25, and DEAE-cellulose column used in tandem. For the cellulose column the remainder of the DEAE-cellulose prepared above is used. For the Sephadex column about half as much bedding as for the DEAE-column is used. The Sephadex has been swelled in 0.01 M phosphate buffer, pH 7.5, for about three hours at room temperature, washed and decanted in this buffer several times and deaerated at 1–5° overnight under avoidance of stirring. It has been poured into the

Fig. 2-5 Separation of optimally conjugated fluorescein-labeled IgG from crude conjugate by G-25 and DEAE cellulose columns used in tandem. R, reservoir containing 0.01 M phosphate buffer, pH 7.5 (I); G, gradient reservoir equipped with stirrer containing 0.01 M phosphate buffer, pH 7.5 on one side (I); and 0.1 M phosphate buffer, pH 7.5 in 0.5 M sodium chloride solution on the other side (II). Both sides are connected with a valve. T, T-tube; Pl, plunger; P, chromatography pump; S, flow spectrometer; C, conductivity bridge; F, fraction collector.

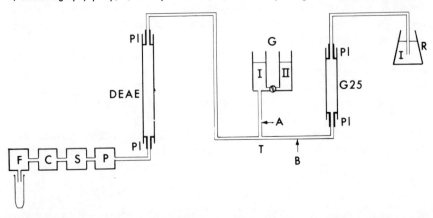

column under gentle agitation with a stirrer suspended into the filling funnel. Preparation of the columns is to be completed prior to conjugation of the IgG with FITC.

Both columns (Fig. 2-5, G25 and DEAE) are connected via two limbs of a T tube (T). The third limb of the T tube is connected to a gradient reservoir (G), containing on one side (I) 0.01 M phosphate buffer, pH 7.5, as the starting buffer and on the other side (II) 0.1 M phosphate buffer, pH 7.5, in 0.5 N sodium chloride solution as gradient forming buffer. Any air bubble that might develop during the connecting of both columns is allowed to escape via the T tube into the buffer reservoir. Liquid can be pushed into this direction by compressing one column with the column plunger (Pl) and leaving access to the other column and to reservoir R closed with clamps. The Sephadex column is connected to a reservoir containing starting buffer (I). The free end of the DEAE cellulose column is connected to the fraction collector, preferably, via a dual wavelength recording flow spectrometer and a conductivity bridge.

Continuing work at 1–5°, both columns are equilibriated with starting buffer (I) from the reservior (R) on the Sephadex column, while the T tube connection with the gradient reservoir remains closed (clamp at A). Equilibriation is assured by equal osmolarity or conductivity of effluent and starting buffer.

The conjugated IgG cleared by centrifugation is applied to the top of the Sephadex column and is followed by starting buffer (0.01 M phosphate pH 7.5). Separation of the leading fluorescent conjugate from the trailing free fluorescein is visibly observed by their yellow-greenish color. As soon as the leading color band has entered the DEAE cellulose column, the Sephadex column is separated from the system by closing its connection with the T tube (clamp B). At the same time the connection of the gradient reservoir (G) and the T tube is opened (clamp A). While the connection between both sides of the gradient reservoir is closed, a volume of starting buffer (I) from the gradient reservoir approximately equal to the volume of the Sephadex column is permitted to flow into the DEAE-cellulose column. Starting buffer is then added to the starting buffer side of the gradient reservoir so that the height of liquid on the starting and the gradient buffer side is equal. Both sides of the reservoir are then connected to initiate gradient elution.

The molar Fl/P ratio, monitored either continuously or on individual fractions by optical density (OD) determinations at 280 and 440 nm, is

$$\frac{(OD_{490} \text{ of conjugate}) \cdot 0.244 \cdot 150{,}000}{\left[(OD_{280} \text{ of conjugate}) - \dfrac{(OD_{490} \text{ of conjugate}) \cdot (OD_{280} \text{ of fluorescein diacetate})}{(OD_{490} \text{ of fluorescein diacetate})}\right] \cdot 0.62 \cdot 374}$$

using a molecular weight of 374 for fluorescein and 150,000 for IgG. Fractions possessing ratios between 1.0 to 1.5 are pooled, concentrated by pressure dialysis, dialyzed against PBS and, following redetermination of the Fl/P ratio, passed through sterile Millipore filters and stored at 1–5° under protection from light.

Although the measured Fl/P ratio does not reflect the accurate proportion of *conjugated* FITC to protein, it is under these conditions of measurement that the apparent ratios of 1.0–1.5 have been established as optimal for immunofluorescence staining.

W. Arnold and H. Von Mayersbach have shown that IgG labeled with fluorescein isothiocyanate forms precipitates on storage irrespective of whether the conjugated protein has been merely dialyzed or passed through Sephadex G25 or in addition through DEAE-cellulose. The extent of precipitation increases with the Fl/P ratio of the conjugate and with decreasing pH. Development of these precipitates decreases nonspecific staining by the remaining supernates. The finding illustrates the source of the most important nonspecific staining in immunofluorescence or in any other immunocytochemical method that uses labeled antibodies, namely the increase in polarity of the IgG molecule as result of conjugation. Nonspecific attachment to tissue surfaces or intermolecular aggregation leading eventually to precipitation are expressions of increased polarity.

Instead of separating from conjugate by DEAE-cellulose chromatography those fractions that possess low Fl/P ratios, Arnold and Von Mayersbach suggest a method that yields as fluorescent conjugate nearly all the antibody activity that has been present in the IgG before conjugation. Essentially, they recommend conjugation in mixtures containing 8–10 mg fluorescein isothiocyanate per gm of IgG in the usual 0.5 M carbonate buffer, pH 9.5, followed by dialysis against 0.01 M phosphate buffer, pH 6.8, for 3–6 days at 4°. (The lowered pH enhances time-dependent precipitation.) Following centrifugation at 10,000 g for 20 minutes, the supernate is readjusted by passage through Sephadex G25 equilibriated with phosphate buffer 0.01 M, pH 7.5, in phosphate and 0.15 M in sodium chloride. Nonspecific fluorescence of the product should be checked, and if still present the pH for precipitation may be lowered slightly.

PURIFIED CONJUGATED ANTIBODIES

Often it would appear that the use of purified antibodies (purified *after* conjugation) would have several advantages over chromatographic isolation of IgG and chromatographic separation of optimal conjugate, each followed by time-consuming concentrations. First, purified antibody is immunologically more specific than isolated IgG, which contains all the

IgG antibodies produced by an immune animal and not only those of desired immunologic specificity. Second, purification by immunoabsorption does not dilute the antibodies. Indeed, antibody elution from an immunoabsorbent can be done in such a manner as to increase the concentration of specific antibody over that of the starting material. Third, immunoabsorption is as efficient as chromatography in separating free fluorescein from conjugate. Fourth, immunoabsorbents can be used to exchange the carbonate buffer used in conjugation with PBS or other buffers used in staining. Fifth, and most important, immunoabsorption eliminates automatically that portion of antibody that has been destroyed during conjugation with FITC.

There are, however, two drawbacks in the purification that have prevented its extensive use in immunofluorescence. First, specific purification does not separate unconjugated antibody, conjugated antibody having an optimal Fl/P ratio and antibodies having higher Fl/P ratios but still possessing antibody activity. Second, immunoabsorbents while yielding proteins that are nearly 100% specific antibody seldom release the purified antibodies in yields higher than 70% on single elution (yield varies with nature of antigen, avidity of antibody, and degree of saturation of the immunoabsorbent, page 15). In some, but not all antigen-antibody systems, the antibody that is released from the immunoabsorbent is that fraction of total antibody with the lowest avidity and, hence, highest cross-reactivity with nonspecific antigenic determinants. In immunohistochemical staining it is important that the antibody is firmly bound to tissue and is not removed during the necessary washing procedures. Purified antibody when it is of low avidity has an increased chance of being lost during washing. On the other hand, under special conditions immunoabsorbents could also be used for enhancing the specific binding quality of antibodies. If a large excess of antiserum relative to the capacity of the immunoabsorbent is used, antibodies with higher binding avidity will be selected by the immunoabsorbent. It will be necessary, however, in a preliminary test to ascertain that the antibody absorbed under these conditions can be eluted from the immunoabsorbent efficiently.

Just as tissues exhibit nonspecific reactions with those portions of conjugate that contain excessive amounts of FITC, so does the immunoabsorbent. Fortunately, such nonspecifically absorbed protein is less efficiently eluted by acid treatment than the specifically bound antibody. Indeed, conjugated antibodies eluted from immunoabsorbents possess lower Fl/P ratios than those of the immunoglobulin applied.

One percent homologous normal serum protein should be added to purified, conjugated antibody preparations if stored at 0–6°. The preparations have to be passed through a bacterial filter unless used immediately. Alternatively, preparations can be quick frozen in dry ice and acetone and stored below −20°. After lyophilization, difficulties have been encountered in redissolving conjugates of purified antibody or of immunoglobulin.

Tissue Preparation

Free, noncontiguous cells, such as bacteria, or protozoa, or blood cells, or free floating cells obtained from reticuloendothelial organs or cells dissociated from tissue culture monolayers, can be stained without sectioning either in suspension or on smears placed on glass slides. If a suspended cell is *living,* only antigens on the cell membrane accept specific immunofluorescence because antibodies do not passively penetrate the interior of living cells. Antibodies do, however, enter occasional living cells by pinocytosis. Conjugated immunoglobulin so imbibed will not be passively released upon washing. Hence, the interior of living cells while normally remaining unstained may occasionally become nonspecifically stained. Specific staining in fluorescence microscopy appears as fluorescent rings that outline the cell surface if the antigen is widely distributed on the cell surface (Fig. 8–6). Granular or patchy staining should be interpreted with caution (page 103). On living cells transplantation (H2) isoantigens have been identified in normal and malignant mouse cells, tumor specific antibodies on cultured Burkitt lymphoma cells and Ig (receptor) determinants on the surface of mouse lymphoid cells (page 194). Viability tests are carried out prior to staining because unfixed, dead cells are penetrable to antibodies and stain nonspecifically.

When making smears of free cells on glass slides for observation of nonliving cells, it is usually desirable to cover the glass slides with a protein solution in order to insure adherence of the applied cells during the staining and washing procedure. Allowing slides to dry spontaneously after application of a 0.1% solution of gelatin or serum albumin is usually satisfactory. Cells are applied either by spreading the suspension on the slide or by placement of drops of dilute suspension on the surface of the slide. The slides are then treated with a suitable fixative solution, a procedure that helps penetration of antibodies to the interior of the cells, assures cell death and, thus, prevents pinocytosis, aids the adherence of the cells to the slide via the intervening gelatin or protein layer, and may suppress nonspecific staining of cells that may have been dead prior to fixation.

Solid tissue, in contrast to free cells, must be sectioned to avoid scattering of image-forming light. For light microscopy at a resolution of 2 μ, interference of tissue overlaying the focal plane is minimal if the thickness of the section is less than that of an average tissue cell. Sections of 2–6 μ thickness, more or less, are suitable for immunofluorescence microscopy.

Staining for fluorescence microscopy of solid tissue is done on the section. As the thickness of the section is less than that of the cells, the cells are cut open, making their interior readily accessible to antibodies.

Fresh tissues are not rigid enough to be sectioned by the microtome. To facilitate sectioning, tissues must either be frozen or infiltrated with paraffin. The choice of procedure depends on the antigen to be studied.

Frozen sections are prepared in the freezing microtome, thawed after application to glass slides and then stained. The procedure is most suitable for insoluble antigens that do not become dislocated during staining and washing. Instead of frozen sections of 2–6 μ thickness, a tissue chopper can be used and 20–30 μ thick sections again be stained without fixation. For soluble antigens frozen sections should be fixed upon thawing. There is some danger of dislocating antigens during fixation because in highly soluble antigens diffusion is more rapid than fixation. This problem is especially severe with formaldehyde fixation, which is slow, but is not very serious with alcohol or acetone precipitation, which is rapid. Perhaps this is one of the reasons why formaldehyde fixation has found rather little application in early immunofluorescence work, although, it is known that the activity of many antigens, such as determinants in diphtheria toxin, are not affected by extensive treatment with formaldehyde. When a soluble antigen is contained within a membrane, such as a lysosomal membrane, it is only necessary to coagulate the membrane in order to contain most of the antigen inside. While fixation in itself makes the membrane sluggishly penetrable to protein, this process is too slow to release the entire contents of a lysosome (exchange of protein through such "fixed" membranes is incomplete even after hours of exposure as will be discussed in connection with antibody penetrability of cells on pages 69 and 123). However, when a soluble antigen held in the intercellular space or within the cytoplasm of a cell opened by sectioning is to be localized, it cannot be contained by coagulation of a surrounding membrane. Instead, the antigen itself must be precipitated irreversibly. This cannot be accomplished by acetone or alcohol on tissue chopper or frozen sections. Instead, the tissue must be fixed, dehydrated by alcohols and embedded in paraffin. Following sectioning and prior to staining, the paraffin must be removed by solvents such as xylene. The procedure is only suitable for antigens withstanding the fixation and the removal of embedding medium. The fixative used must irreversibly precipitate the antigen without destroying its antigenic determinants.

A freeze substitution technique as introduced by R. Post may reduce diffusion artifacts often encountered in the localization of soluble antigen. As used by V. E. Pollak, B. S. Ooi, and A. G. Pesce for the localization of serum albumin in renal biopsy specimens, 1 mm cubes of tissue are frozen in liquid nitrogen, transferred to acetone at −65°, substituted with mixtures of increasing proportions of tetrahydrofuran and acetone, and sectioned 0.5 μ thick at -5 to $-10°$. The ribbon of sections is picked up on a slide previously dipped in potassium chromealum solution to insure adherence.

Once a fixative has been found that does not *abolish* all specific reactivity of the particular antigen under study, it should be used at the highest possible concentration in order to assure optimal preservation of structure and minimal dislocation of soluble antigen.

Fixatives harden tissue because they reduce the solubility of its constituents. This is effected by intermolecular bridges that may be formed by various mechansims:

1. Covalent as with bifunctional aldehydes such as glutaraldehyde.

2. Chelation of a heavy metal such as osmium with two adjacent protein molecules.

3. Precipitation because of reduction of charge and increase in hydrophobicity as with formaldehyde, mercuric chloride, or picric acid.

4. Precipitation because of removal of water as with acetone, or ethanol, or acid-ethanol mixtures (denaturation upon rehydration may be a contributing factor).

5. Unfolding of peptide chains of adjacent protein molecules and entanglement upon refolding such as in denaturation by heat.

Among these fixatives the dehydrants (ethanol, methanol, isopropanol, and acetone) have found widest application in immunocytochemistry because their effect on antigenic reactivity is minimal. Judicious use of formaldehyde (2% formaldehyde freshly prepared from paraformaldehyde at 4°) and more rarely glutaraldehyde can be tolerated by some protein antigens. Polysaccharides and some small molecular proteins, such as pituitary hormones or lysozyme, are more resistant and tolerate high concentrations of aldehydes. Pancreatic enzymes have withstood mixtures of equal parts of dioxane and 30% formaldehyde. Mercuric chloride and osmium tetroxide fixation tend to quench fluorescence.

Let us detail tissue preparation for localization of three types of antigens:

(a) An insoluble antigen illustrated by connective tissue antigen in the work of D. C. Scott.

(b) Soluble antigens that appear at the resolution of immunofluorescence as indiscriminately cytoplasmic but are actually contained within the confines of lysosomes, as is illustrated in the work of S. Morikawa in the localization of ribonuclease in the zymogen granules of the acinar cells of pancreas (an acinus is a grape-like cluster of epithelial cells surrounding a lumen).

(c) A highly soluble protein illustrated by α-fetoprotein in liver cells in the work of N. V. Engelhardt and co-workers using a technique introduced by Sainte-Marie.

Insoluble antigen

Blocks of tissue are quick frozen and sectioned at 4 μ thickness in a cryostat at -18 to $-23°$. The sections are transferred onto glass slides and thawed into position by touching the underside of the slides with an ungloved finger. Use of clean glass assures adherence of the section during staining even without fixation, unless staining times are excessively prolonged.

Antigen confined within membranes

Tissue is fixed by immersion into dry ice and acetone. 3 to 4 μ thick sections are cut at $-20°$, thawed onto clean glass slides, and allowed to dry at room temperature for 15 minutes. The sections are then fixed either in 95% ethanol for 30 minutes or in 10% formalin in PBS for 15 minutes. After washing, the sections are stained with FITC-conjugated immunoglobulin.

Soluble antigen

Alpha fetoprotein is found in sera of normal embryos, in adult animals bearing primary or transplanted hepatomas and in patients with hepatocellular carcinoma or with malignant teratoplastoma of testis or ovary. For the localization of α-fetoprotein by immunofluorescence 3 × 4 × 5 mm specimens of mouse or human fetal liver and of biopsy material from patients with primary hepatic carcinoma are fixed at 0–6° in 95% ethanol containing 1% glacial acetic acid. Following hardening by the fixative for one hour, the tissue blocks are trimmed so as to have at least one flat surface and then returned to the fixative for 15–24 hours. They are dehydrated in four changes of absolute ethanol for a total of 20 minutes, keeping the blocks sufficiently agitated so that their floating above the bottom of the container accelerates dehydration. The blocks are cleared by four changes of xylene for a total of 20 minutes at 0–6° and then allowed to come to room temperature while still in xylene. They are embedded by passage through four 1–2 hour changes of paraffin at 56°. They are sectioned soon after embedding to minimize autofluorescence.

Three micron thick sections are floated on water at 40° and mounted on clean glass slides without adhesives, removing excess fluid with a filter paper. The sections are deparaffinized in two changes of xylene at 0–6° for 10–15 minutes each, keeping the slides in continuous up-and-down motion with care to avoid dislocation of the section. The xylene is then removed by a similar procedure in three changes of 95% ethanol and the ethanol in turn by three changes of Tris buffer pH 7.2.

Staining

Immunocytochemistry depends on the primary binding of antibodies (page 7) and not on secondary effects of the bound antibody. Consequently, antibodies of any immunoglobulin class or even monovalent fragments of antibodies (page 6) are suitable reagents. The fact that binding has occurred is detected by separation of the specifically bound fluorescent antibody from unbound fluorescent material. The separation depends on two requirements: the tissue component to be stained must remain insoluble during the staining procedure (hence, the need for adequate fixation for all but insoluble antigens) and the immunocytochemical reagents must be highly soluble (free from aggregated material and material of borderline solubilities that can be insolubilized by the tissue nonspecifically.) In principle, staining consists of application of a solution containing specific antibody that results in binding of that specific antibody, leaving all nonspecific components of the IgG and of other proteins in solution. These nonspecific components are removed by washing. The entirety of precautions necessary for immunocytochemical specificity depends on assuring that during staining specific antibody is the only component that changes phase.

There are several staining sequences for localization of the antigen-antibody reaction in tissues by fluorescence:

1. *Direct technique:* Tissue antigen binds FITC-labeled specific antibody.

2. *Indirect technique:* In the first step tissue antigen binds specific unlabeled antibody from species "a." In a second step the bound unlabeled antibody binds FITC-labeled antibody to the immunoglobulin of species "a" produced in species "b."

3. *Complement technique:* In the first step tissue antigen binds specific antibody (IgG or IgM). In the second step complement is applied in the form of guinea pig serum in the presence of calcium and magnesium ions. In the third step FITC-conjugated immunoglobulin antiguinea pig complement is bound.

4. *Staining of intracellular antibody:* Detection of intracellular antibody simply by addition of fluorescein-conjugated specific antigen is not a very sensitive method. In the more commonly used procedure, tissue is first reacted with unlabeled specific antigen followed by FITC-labeled antibody to this antigen.

5. *Double staining technique:* Antigen "a" stains green by binding antibody from FITC-labeled anti-"a," and antigen "b" in the same tissue stains orange-red by binding antibody from lissamine rhodamine B200 labeled anti-"b."

6. *Sequential technique:* In the first step antigen "a" binds fluorescein-labeled anti-"a." The staining pattern is recorded photographically. The fluorescence is destroyed by prolonged exposure to the full beam of ultraviolet light. In the second step a second antigen "b" is localized with fluorescein-labeled anti-"b" and the finding recorded photographically.

Staining is usually done at room temperature, and the slides are kept in a humid chamber, such as a large Petri dish equipped with a moistened beaker mat. Reagents are most commonly applied for 30 minutes, but much variation in application time is possible. Following each reagent, the slides are rinsed first with a stream of buffer and then placed usually for five minutes in a jar containing buffer. PBS, pH 7.0, or saline containing 0.05 M Tris buffer pH 7.0–7.6 are most commonly used, but many other buffers in this pH range are satisfactory. If tissues have been fixed with aldehydes, especially glutaraldehyde, Tris buffer appears to reduce nonspecific staining as compared to phosphate buffer. Conceivably, the Tris buffer reacts with any free aldehyde groups remaining in the tissue and competes, thereby, for these groups with the protein of the staining reagent. The use of sodium bisulfite for treatment of aldehyde-fixed tissue prior to staining does not reduce nonspecific reactivity, apparently because of insufficient concentration of both the bisulfite as well as the unreacted aldehyde groups.

To mount sections, a cover slip is placed on a piece of filter paper, a drop of polyvinyl alcohol is put on the cover slip, the slide with the section is inverted, and the section is allowed to touch the drop. To squeeze out excess mounting medium, the slide is then pressed onto the cover slip, gently avoiding lateral motion that could displace or distort the section. The cover slip is sealed around the edges with nail polish.

Direct technique

A fluorescent antibody preparation is needed for each antigen to be localized. The procedure is, therefore, only convenient if a large amount of antiserum is available and if many preparations are to be examined for the same antigen. As the procedure only involves a single antibody prep-

aration, nonspecific reaction is minimized. The direct technique is typi-
cally, but not exclusively used in the study of autoimmune disease (Chapter 9) in which labeled antiimmunoglobulin is applied to tissues containing
antigen-antibody complexes.

Indirect technique

This is the most widely used technique because a single preparation
of labeled anti-IgG can be used for detection of antibodies of different
specificities from a single species. For most applications labeled anti-IgG
rather than antibodies against other classes of immunoglobulin are used
because IgG is the most abundant and most easily prepared class of immunoglobulins, because most antibodies in hyperimmune sera used in the
first step are of IgG class, and because the L-chains of IgG are identical
with those of other classes.

Since IgG possesses a number of antigenic determinants, several anti-
IgG molecules applied in the second step can react with a single antibody
molecule bound in the first step. This increases the sensitivity of the indirect method about 10-fold as compared to that of the direct method.
However, part of the increase in sensitivity may be due to the fact that
anti-IgG sera usually are hyperimmune sera containing a larger amount
of antibody than antisera used in the direct method and that hyperimmune
antibodies usually possess higher avidities.

The unlabeled antibody in the indirect method should be applied in
the form of antiserum. Immunoglobulin prepared from antisera is contra-
indicated unless the preparations have been high speed centrifuged to
remove any aggregated material. Otherwise, aggregated material left in
the immunoglobulin fraction would adhere to tissue nonspecifically and
react with the subsequently applied FITC-anti-IgG. There is no advantage
in using Ig or IgG rather than immune serum in the first step, since in both
cases nonrelevant protein is removed by washing with equal ease. Purified
antibody is indicated only if the procedure renders antibody monospecific
to a particular tissue component by separating the antibody from serum
that also contains antibodies to other components.

Immunofluorescence is not only used for the detection of antigens in
tissues, but also diagnostically for the determination of antibody titers in
sera. An example is the diagnosis of syphilitic infection by titration of
patient's antiserum with treponemal suspensions, followed by indirect immunofluorescence using FITC-conjugated goat antihuman immunoglobulin. A semi-quantitative titer is obtained by determining the dilution of the
patient's serum in which immunofluorescence is no longer clearly apparent.
In a direct method the titer would only depend on the patient's serum
dilution. In the indirect method, however, the titer depends on the dilution

of the patient's serum as well as on the dilution of the fluorescent immuno-globulin. Theoretically, this difficulty could be avoided by using a large excess of antiimmunoglobulin so that the reaction of the second step will be first order in the patient's antibodies. Unfortunately, high concentrations of conjugated antibodies cannot be used because they foster nonspecific reactions. (This illustrates one of the main problems encountered with any immunocytochemical method that uses labeled antibodies, whatever the nature of the label. Herein lies the main reason for using only un-labeled antibodies in the development of molecular immunocytochemistry discussed in Chapter 7.) In order to compare antibody titers from different patients, it is desirable, therefore, to use a large pool of the same prepara-tion of fluorescent anti-IgG. As fluorescent immunoglobulin is not stable beyond one year, it is also convenient to have available a standard human antiserum that can be divided into small portions and quick frozen in-definitely. A new batch of fluorescent anti-IgG can then be calibrated by titration (Table 2–1) and used at a concentration that gives the same titer of standard serum as the previous anti-IgG preparation.

The alternative approach to standardization, namely that of defining the properties of FITC-conjugated anti-IgG sufficiently to give predictable titers with standard first step antisera, has not been possible because it requires (1) a predictable Fl/P ratio of the conjugate, (2) a predictable amount of antibody remaining immunologically active after conjugation,

Table 2-1

Immunofluorescence of *T. pallidum*, titrated with dilutions of serum of a syphilitic patient and fluorescein-conjugated goat immunoglobulin antihuman IgG

Antiglobulin dilutions	Patient's serum dilutions						
	5 *	10	20	40	80	160	320
10 *	++++	++++	+++	++	+	±	—
20	++++	++++	+++	++	+	±	—
40	++++	++++	+++	++	+	±	—
80	++++	++++	+++	++	+	±	—
160	++++	+++	++	++	—	—	—
360	+++	++	+	—	—	—	—
1280	+	±	—	—	—	—	—
2560	—	—	—	—	—	—	—
5120	—	—	—	—	—	—	—

The end points (heavy lines on the chessboard titration) did not only depend on the concentration of the patient's serum, but also on that of the fluorescent conjugate. (From the work of P. H. Hardy and E. E. Nell. *Am. J. Clin. Path.*, **56**:181, 1971.)

* Reciprocal of dilutions

(3) predictable retention of activity upon storage, and (4) predictable avidities. While the first three factors can conceivably be controlled, heterogeneity of antibodies—evoked by the same antigen in different animals and in the same animals at varying time intervals during immunization—introduces variability in avidity of the anti-IgG conjugates, even when the Fl/P ratio and the *amount* of antibody are kept constant.

Complement technique

This three step method usually uses guinea pig serum as a source of complement. The binding of complement is evaluated by fluorescein-conjugated immunoglobulin containing antibodies to guinea pig complement. Since guinea pig complement is bound by IgM and aggregated IgG of any mammalian source, the same antiguinea pig complement can be used for analysis of localization of antibodies from different mammalian sources. This permits, for example, comparison of immunofluorescence titers of human and rabbit antisyphilitic sera. Such a comparison would have been difficult with the indirect method that would require both a fluorescein-conjugated antihuman and a fluorescein-conjugated antirabbit IgG. The immunofluorescence potencies of these anti-IgG's cannot be compared since they cannot be titered with the same standard antisyphilitic serum.

Unlike other immunocytochemical techniques, the complement technique is a primary binding technique only in the first and third step. The second step depends on the ability of the bound immunoglobulin to fix complement. Only IgM and IgG fix complement. A single antigen site binding a single IgM molecule suffices. IgG, however, must be aggregated at least to the size of a dimer in order to fix complement. Hence, IgG after reaction with a cell surface will only fix complement if its concentration has been sufficiently high so as to bind onto two adjacent antigen sites, thus bringing two IgG molecules into direct apposition. If antigen is in excess (weak or diluted antiserum), the chance of occurrence of such juxtaposition becomes small. Hence, for sera containing IgG, but devoid of IgM, the three step complement test can only be used with relatively high serum concentrations. High concentrations of sera reduce, however, the specificity of immunofluorescence.

The complement method can conceivably be used to differentiate between IgM and IgG antibodies, when the titers obtained by the three-step procedure are compared with a four-step procedure, such as the following: in the first step, antiserum from species "a" specific for the tissue antigen is applied; in the second step, sheep serum anti-"a" IgG is used; in the third step, guinea pig complement is applied; and in the fourth step, FITC-conjugated rabbit immunoglobulin anti-guinea pig complement that has been absorbed with normal sheep serum. Titers are determined by the maximum dilution of the antiserum applied in the first step which yields barely discernible fluorescence. If the first-step antibodies are IgM, the four-step procedure would increase the titer slightly when compared to the three-step procedure. However, if the first-step antibodies are IgG, titers would increase markedly, an increase beyond 20-fold probably being significant. This is so because, at limiting antiserum dilutions at which in the three-step test fluorescence is barely visible, only rare IgG antibodies bind to adjacent antigen sites. However, when sheep serum anti-IgG is added, each singly bound IgG molecule from the serum of the first step becomes complexed with several sheep IgG molecules and hence, capable of binding complement.

Antisera to complement are conveniently produced in rabbits by injection of washed immune precipitates produced by interaction of BSA, rabbit serum anti-BSA heated to 56° for 30 minutes, and fresh guinea pig serum. The use of rabbit immune precipitates for immunization of rabbits minimizes the amount of anti-IgG produced. However, it will be necessary to absorb the anticomplement sera with the sera from the BSA-immunized rabbits if one wants to be sure that immunofluorescence is only due to the complement test and is devoid of an indirect immunofluorescence component due to alloantibodies (antiimmunoglobulins specific to genetic immunoglobulin markers unshared among the immunoglobulins of the anti-BSA and the antiimmune precipitate rabbits). The anticomplement sera react predominantly with C3.

Alternative methods preclude the formation of alloantibodies. Thus, instead of immune precipitates, aggregated IgG from the rabbit to be immunized, or from an allotypically homozygous rabbit may be used for fixation of guinea pig complement. Also, instead of immune precipitates, complement components could be used for immunization of rabbits.

Clq is bound at the site of interaction of antibody with antigen. C3, however, has been shown by immunocytochemistry both with the immuno-ferritin (page 73) and the unlabeled antibody enzyme method (page 158) to be bound over a wide area of contiguity on a cell surface, even when the antigen-antibody sites are discrete and widely dispersed. Hence, the complement method when it utilizes anti-C3 does not delineate the sites of antigen-antibody interaction at subcellular dimensions. The method cannot be used at resolutions higher than that of identifying reacting cells and gives incorrect localization when adapted to electron microscopic immunocytochemistry.

Staining of intracellular antibody

Since macromolecular antigens usually possess a number of antigenic determinants, application to tissue of specific antigen followed by fluorescein-labeled antibody attaches a number of fluorescent antibody molecules to each reacting tissue antibody site and affords, thereby, a degree of amplification. For instance, in the production of antidinitrophenyl (anti-DNP) antibody, DNP-hemocyanin is injected into a mouse. Spleen cells producing anti-DNP are reacted first with DNP-human serum albumin (HSA) containing about 20 DNP groups per molecule. Several of these 20 groups, perhaps as much as ⅓ of them, can react with subsequently applied fluorescein-conjugated anti-DNP-hemocyanin (HSA does not cross-react with hemocyanin and hence, only the cells producing anti-DNP and not those producing antihemocyanin will be localized). It has been found empirically that detection of antibodies is further improved if the section is refixed in 95% ethanol for 15 minutes at 0–6° after application of the antigen and the usual buffer wash and prior to application of fluorescein-conjugated antibody. The ethanol is removed by three rinses in buffer at room temperature for one minute each. A similar post-fixation is thought to improve the preservation of stained slides after application of fluorescein-conjugated antibody and prior to mounting. Conceivably, the refixation and postfixation prevent slow dissociation of antibody from antigen in subsequently applied media. While the reaction of most antibodies with antigen is rapid and the reverse reaction slow, dissociation does occur and is favored by extensive washing, rise in temperature, and prolongation of subsequent staining steps. Qualitative evaluation of dissociation by immunofluorescence and quantitative evaluation by the unlabeled antibody enzyme method are described on pages 51 and 176.

Double-staining technique

Both fluorescein and rhodamine-conjugated antibodies must be used by direct technique. They may be applied in a single mixture. The technique is useful for the simultaneous detection by contrasting colors (green and orange-red) of two antigens in different cells of the same section. Two antigens in the same cell are detected by intermediate colors (mixed fluorescence), such as yellow or orange, provided the two conjugates are strictly specific to the antigens without cross-reaction. The double-staining technique can also be utilized to demonstrate monospecificity of antibodies produced by a single cell (page 199). When fluorescein and rhodamine-conjugated antibodies are applied sequentially, the technique can be used to measure degrees of cross-reactivity of two different antisera with the same antigen in a cell. Finally, on sequential incubation, the technique can give an estimate of the degree of dissociation of tissue-bound antibody during subsequent incubation (page 51).

Sequential technique

Nash, Crabbé, and Heremans used sequential staining of plasma cells from mice immunized with ferritin to determine for each cell the class of immunoglobulin produced and to establish which immunoglobulin-containing cell produces immunoglobulin with specificity for ferritin. Sections were treated with ferritin followed by fluorescein-conjugated rabbit IgG antiferritin. After mounting the sections, the cells were photographed. Prints were made by projecting the negative image through a lattice of

Fig. 2-6 In sequential immunofluorescence staining of cells from the lymphoid tissue of a mouse immunized with ferritin, the antiferritin producing cells are identified and located upon a grid of coordinates (F-AF). Fluorescence is then destroyed by ultraviolet irradiation (IR), and cells producing IgA are localized (A) on the same coordinates. The cell marked by the arrow does not appear in frame F-AF. Hence, this cell contains IgA of specificity other than antiferritin. After application of fluorescein-conjugated anti-IgM, the IgA containing cell is still seen in addition to a fair number of IgM containing cells (AM). The cells denoted by the arrows also appear in frame F-AF. Hence, they contain IgM antiferritin. However, the large cells in grid location B3 and B4 do not appear in frame F-AF and contain, therefore, IgM not reactive with ferritin. Most of the IgG_1 containing cells (frame AMG_1) also appear in frame F-AF, except those marked by arrows that seem to contain IgG of specificities other than antiferritin. Staining with anti-IgG_2 added only few cells (AMG_1G_2, arrows). Their IgG_2 is specific for ferritin.

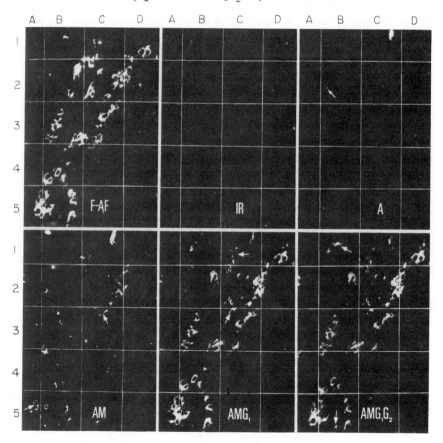

coordinates made by stretching silk screens across the masking frame of the photographic paper (Fig. 2-6 FAF). The photographed section was kept in place in the fluorescent microscope and exposed upon removal of all filters to the full ultraviolet beam for 10 to 20 minutes. Extinction of all fluorescence is confirmed in Fig. 2-6 IR. The cover slip was gently removed from the slide by immersion into buffer. The section was then incubated with fluorescein-labeled anti-IgA and photographed. A print was made by aligning the negative in the same position over the coordinates as the previous print (Fig. 2-6 A). Without further ultraviolet irradiation, the cover slip was removed, and the section exposed to fluorescein-conjugated rabbit IgG antimouse IgM. The procedure was then repeated with anti-IgG$_1$ and anti-IgG$_2$ in sequence (Fig. 2-6 AM, AMG$_1$, and AMG$_1$G$_2$).

Serial sectioning and exposure of each section to specific antibodies can provide answers similar to the sequential technique. However, serial sectioning often leaves doubt as to whether the same cell is being examined particularly since immunofluorescence does not reveal much morphology besides the spots, or rings, or clusters that fluoresce. The double-staining technique that addresses itself to similar problems as the sequential technique sometimes encounters difficulties in interpretation of colors resulting from mixtures of green and orange-red when both antibodies react in the same cell.

Other staining combinations

Nonimmunologic staining techniques can be employed to obtain morphologic information beyond that possible by dark field immunofluorescence. These techniques are always applied after immunofluorescence staining and photography of the immunofluorescence observations because nonimmunologic staining reagents are liable to impair tissue antigens and because many of the stains (such as eosin) are in themselves fluorescent.

MICROSCOPY AND PHOTOGRAPHY

Specific fluorescence emission is relatively weak compared to the total light necessary for illumination. Therefore, high intensity light as provided by the mercury arc high vacuum lamp is necessary to obtain bright immunofluorescence.

Although fluorescein and rhodamine absorb strongly below 300 nm, optical difficulties of condensing light in this range preclude its routine use. A second absorption maximum for these fluorochromes is too near the emission peak: fluorescence microscopy is sensitive because the emitted light is seen against a dark background. To this end, it is important that only the emitted light is seen and not the illuminating light. Since only part of the illuminating light becomes absorbed, the unabsorbed part must be separated from the emitted light. This separation cannot be accomplished if both illuminating and emitted light have close peaks. Hence, for immunofluorescence with rhodamine and fluorescein, illuminating light in the near ultraviolet and short wave blue are used. In this range, both fluorescein and rhodamine absorb though not as efficiently as at shorter or longer wavelengths. Filters, such as Schott BG12, placed between light source and specimen, will provide this range of light. A BG38 filter is added for protection. To retain only the fluorescence emission light, additional filters must be placed between specimen and ocular. The filter should absorb the light passed by the BG12 filter (the illuminating light used), without interfering with the fluorescence emission light. K-510 ocular filters or OG1 + CG9 filters have been used.

With judicious use of filters, it is possible to obtain bright field fluorescence and still observe fluorescence emission under complete exclusion of illuminating light. However, dark field illumination greatly simplifies the selection of filters, since even without filters it insures that most of the illuminating light will not reach the ocular, and that only the fluorescence emission light is seen. In practice dark field condensers are commonly used in conjunction with the above named filters. Glycerine is used in place of an immersion oil for studies of immunofluorescence under immersion lenses.

Photography is essential as fluorescence wanes on storage of specimens. This decrease in fluorescence intensity is also an important factor in the technique of photography itself: total light intensity is often low in dark-field microscopy, especially when only a small part of the section is immunofluorescent. Hence, exposure times tend to be long. However, during long exposure time, fluorescence intensity itself fades. Consequently, attempts should be made to use shortest possible exposure times; therefore, films with high ASA ratings are recommended. Furthermore, a well standardized automatic exposure meter is necessary because light measurement is synchronized with the exposure, and any decrease of fluorescence during exposure is automatically compensated for.

SPECIFICITY

Immunocytochemistry requires two-fold specificity: the antibodies used must be specific for the antigens under investigation, and the immunocytochemical reagents should not stain tissues by mechanisms other than immunologic reactions. We will call nonspecificity of the former class "antibody nonspecificity" and nonspecificity of the latter class "staining nonspecificity."

Staining nonspecificity

Electrostatic and hydrophobic bonding of staining reagents with tissue are the chief causes of staining nonspecificity. When hydrophobic bonding increases, protein tends to aggregate. The macromolecular complexes formed as a result of protein aggregation have a greater tendency than monomeric protein to bind tissue nonspecifically. Aggregation is promoted by removal of water from protein, such as in salt fractionation, or by reaction with polar substituents, as in the conjugation of isothiocyanate with protein amine. Partial insolubilization during conjugation are symptoms of excessive aggregation. Oligomeric protein aggregates will not cloud the solution. Examples of nonspecific staining by such oligomeric aggregates are encountered in the use of ammonium sulfate-precipitated immunoglobulin instead of whole serum in the first step of the indirect immunofluorescence reaction. High-speed centrifugation clears solutions of oligomeric aggregates. The selection of immunofluorescent conjugates of low Fl/P ratio mitigates against inclusion of aggregated material in the conjugate. Herein lies the reason that staining nonspecificity in immunofluorescence is less serious than that of other conjugated antibody methods (pages 83 and 115).

A further factor in staining nonspecificity is electrostatic attraction or salt linkage investigated in detail by H. Von Mayersbach. A net positive charge of tissue relative to that of immunoglobulin increases nonspecific staining. Cytoplasm that is acidophilic exhibits, therefore, varying degrees of nonspecific staining while nuclei that are basophilic do not. Formaldehyde fixation, though not always suitable for immunofluorescence, decreases nonspecific staining by blockage of amino groups and increase of negative charge. In contrast, necrotic tissue or dead cells in suspension exhibit increased nonspecific staining. In the conjugation, increase of negative charge of antibodies increases nonspecificity, but judicious use of conjugates of low Fl/P ratio minimizes this factor.

Fortunately, the nonspecific reaction is rarely of similar order of magnitude as the specific reaction. Thus, in rabbits infected with *Treponema pallidum* the specific indirect immunofluorescence titers range usually between 1:320 to 1:1,280. The nonspecific titer with normal serum is about 1:10. If the conjugated antiimmunoglobulin is of low titer, the specific titer decreases, but the nonspecific titer still is 1:10. For this reason, it is important to use conjugates with high antibody activity. Conjugation always entails some loss of antibody activity. However, in immunofluorescence the loss of antibody activity is less than that encountered in some other immunocytochemical methods that employ covalently conjugated antibodies, because in immunofluorescence, the conjugation reaction is a single-step reaction between conjugant and protein that can be controlled to yield products of low conjugant-protein ratio. Also, FITC is a small molecule compared to immunoglobulin and, therefore, upon mild conjugation the probability of inhibiting antibody activity by steric hindrance remains low.

Antibody nonspecificity

In order of increasing clinical importance, the factors contributing to antibody nonspecificity are as follows:

1. Cross-reactions due to variable region heterogeneity of antibodies.
2. Natural antibodies.
3. Cross-reactions due to multiplicity of antibodies evoked by different types of antigenic determinants in the antigen used for immunization.
4. Cross-reactions due to contamination of the immunizing antigens.
5. Cross-reactions due to unknown antigenic determinants in various tissues.

Variable region heterogeneity

Even antibodies evoked by a defined peptide sequence are heterogeneous in binding with the antigen (heterogeneity of the antibody binding sites page 6). For example, Schechter studied antibodies produced by immunization with poly-L-alanyl human serum albumin (HSA), purified by immunoabsorption with this antigen and elution with tetra-L-alanine. Binding of the antibody with tetra-L-alanine and tetraalanine in which one or more L-alanines was replaced by D-alanine showed that the antibodies were heterogeneous in their combining sites, the majority of molecules only recognizing the N-terminal and pentultimate amino acid. Some antibodies recognized the three terminal alanines, and very few were specific to the sequence of four alanines. If these data were interpolated to any antiprotein antibody, one would assume that the majority of such antibodies would recognize only a sequence of two amino acids, and since there are 21 amino acids, antiprotein antibodies could not in general recognize more than $21^2 = 441$ different antigenic determinants. Hence, cross-reacting would be extensive. In fact, such extensive cross-reactivity has not been observed in immunocytochemistry. Indeed, it is likely that hundreds of thousands of different antiprotein specificities are within the immunocompetence of a normal mammalian host. The explanation of the discrepancy probably lies in the selection of antibodies during purification. By using tetraalanine for elution, only 37% of the polyalanine reactivity and much less of the total antipolyalanyl HSA activity was eluted. It is probable that here—and as we shall see in other applications of immuno-specific purification as well (page 132)—only the antibodies with the lowest binding avidities were eluted, while the highest quality antibodies remained on the immunoabsorbent. These low binding antibodies exhibited strong cross-reactivity due to the fact that by the very purification procedure only antibodies specific to small sequences were selected. The purified antibody may well react with many proteins in any tissue containing two adjacent alanine residues in a suitably accessible position. Nevertheless, such antibodies, though probably present in most immune sera, prove no threat to the specificity of immunofluorescence. Their binding avidity, being weak compared to that of antibodies specific to longer sequences, makes them more easily dissociable from tissue during the washing procedure in immunofluorescence. For this reason, purified antibodies in immunofluorescence may affect sensitivity more than specificity.

Natural antibodies

The first step in antibody production is specific recognition of the antigens by a few lymphocytes that, as a result of selective differentiation, happen to bear on their surfaces immunoglobulin receptors of the required specificity. It is not known whether without antigen injection a very minimal amount of specific antibody production occurs continually so that, in addition to the presence of specific immunoglobulin on the cell, a normal animal also possesses a small amount of specific antibody in circulation. Alternatively, antibodies existing in normal sera could have been induced by unrecognized, prior antigenic stimulation. Such antibodies are called "natural antibodies." Common natural antibodies are the small amounts of antibody to sheep erythrocytes found in most mammals except sheep and the anti-A and -B activities of normal human sera. Such antibodies may interfere with the control in immunofluorescence in which normal serum is substituted for specific antiserum. Use of dilute antisera usually helps to settle the question, as normal serum in contrast to high titered antiserum loses its reactivity at high dilutions. Removal of immunocytochemical reactivity by absorption of the reactivity from normal serum with specific antigen identifies the reactivity as due to natural antibodies.

Multiplicity of antibodies due to different antigenic determinants

Most protein antigens possess different regions that are antigenic. Each antigenic region usually bears different antigenic determinants. Each determinant evokes its own types of antibodies. Some proteins possess, in addition to specific antigenic determinants, determinants shared with

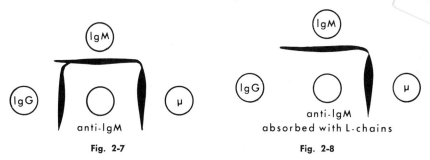

Fig. 2-7

Fig. 2-8

Fig. 2-7 Immunodiffusion of an antiserum specific to an antigen that possesses common determinants with another antigen (schematic). The antiserum (e.g. anti-IgM) forms a single line of identity with its specific antigen (IgM) and a nonspecific antigen (IgG). A second line spurs over this line of identity between the antiserum and the IgM well. This line is due to antibodies that do not precipitate with the IgG and, hence, penetrate its domain until they reach the IgM. Their line of precipitation is confluent with the line of identity, because the antigenic determinants responsible for it are in the same molecule as those responsible for the line of identity. The line of identity between IgM and μ chains is due to the antigenic determinants responsible for this spur.

Fig. 2-8 After absorption of the antiserum (Fig. 2-7) with the determinants shared by the specific antigenic (IgM) and the nonspecifically reacting material (IgG), namely, after absorption with light chains, immunodiffusion has become nonspecific. The line between IgG and the antiserum has disappeared, and only the spuring line of Fig. 2-6 remains (schematic).

other proteins. These shared determinants may lead to nonspecific immunofluorescence. The detection of the class of immunoglobulin contained in an antiferritin-producing cell (Fig. 2-6) requires antisera monospecific for the class. The immunization of rabbits with IgM, for example, yields antibodies specific for IgM that form a single immunodiffusion line and suggests that the IgM used for immunization probably is free of major impurities (Fig. 2-7). However, the antibodies also react with IgG forming a line of identity with IgM. The line of identity is due to antibodies to IgM L-chains that are identical to the IgG L-chains. In addition, however, there is a spur over the line between IgM and the antiserum. This spur is due to antibodies in the antiserum not reactive with IgG. These antibodies penetrate the domain of the diffused IgG without precipitating. They will precipitate only when reaching the fringe of the domain of diffusion of the IgM. These antibodies must be isolated, free of antibody cross-reacting with IgG in order to insure unequivocal localization of the IgM-producing cell (Fig. 2-6 AM). Absorption of the antiserum with L-chains makes it monospecific for IgM (Fig. 2-8).

Cross-reactions due to contamination of the immunizing antigen

When a mixture of antigens is used for immunization, in general most of the antibodies react with the predominant fraction. However, the proportion of antibodies reacting with a minor component to those reacting with a major component is higher in the antiserum than the proportion of minor and major components in the antigen. Thus, the effect of impurities in an antigen preparation is magnified by immunization. Hence, it is common to observe more than one precipitin line when an antiserum against an isolated, presumably purified antigen, is reacted with nonpurified antigen in immunodiffusion. For example, rabbit antiserum to isolated human α-fetoprotein (page 35) gives two precipitin lines with α-fetoprotein-containing adult serum. Removal of one of these lines by absorption with normal adult human serum (devoid of α-fetoprotein) is one of the steps necessary to make the serum monospecific for the diagostic immunocytochemical reaction for primary hepatoma (the other step is separation from antibodies reacting with normal human liver by absorption with and elution from an immunoabsorbent of insolubilized human α-fetoprotein).

Cross-reactions due to unknown antigenic determinants in various tissues

Since immunocytochemistry deals primarily with tissues prior to obtainment of detailed knowledge of all their constituents, this is by far the most common cause of antibody nonspecificity. One does not know to what extent these cross-reactions are due to a multiplicity of antigen molecules in the tissue or tissue fractions used for immunization, some of them also found in other tissues, and to what extent they are due to sharing of similar antigenic determinants among different antigen molecules in different tissues. In either event, different types of antibodies will be formed, some acting with specific tissue only and others reacting with specific as well as nonspecific tissues. In addition, some antibodies may be formed that localize in the specific tissue and in the nonspecific tissue, but the binding of the specific tissue will be stronger. In some cases, as for instance in the reaction of lupus erythematosus autoimmune antisera, it has been possible to isolate the reactive tissue components and to identify the nature of cross-reactions observed with various tissue components and the sera of individual patients. In most cases, however, immunocytochemistry deals with tissue antigens of low solubility that have resisted isolation so far. Nevertheless, distinct steps can be undertaken to make antiserum monospecific to the tissues or cells under investigation. In many cases the efficiency of these steps is best controlled by immunocytochemistry itself. For instance, immunization of rabbits with extracts of beef heart produces autoimmune antibodies reactive by immunofluorescence with sections of rabbit hearts. The reactions are not specific unless the antisera are absorbed with rabbit liver powder (rat or mouse liver is only partially successful).

When a specific unlabeled antiserum is applied to a tissue prior to fluorescein-labeled antibodies, the fluorescence is impaired. If the unlabeled antibodies do not materially dissociate during application of the labeled antibodies, blocking is complete. Blocking can be overcome by increasing the dilution of the unlabeled antibodies, or the concentration of the labeled antibodies, and by increasing the relative time of exposure to labeled antibodies. If the unlabeled antibodies are not homologous to the labeled antibodies, but cross-reactive, blocking is liable to be only partial.

The double-staining technique has been used sequentially by P. E. Scott to study cross-reactive immunofluorescence of rabbit immunoglobulin antihuman glomerulus and rabbit immunoglobulin antihuman synovium. Each immunoglobulin was labeled with fluorescein and rhodamine (RH). When only fluorescein-conjugated antibodies reacted, fluorescence was green. When only rhodamine-conjugated antibodies reacted, fluorescence was orange-red. When one of these antibodies only partially blocked reaction of the second antibody, fluorescence was of intermediate color, namely greenish-yellow, yellow, or orange.

Conjugated antiglomerulus, when preceded only by normal rabbit immunoglobulin, stained in the kidney the glomerular basement membrane, the peritubular capillaries, and the vascular adventitia; it also stained the splenic reticulum and the synovium (Table 2-2, lines 5 and 7). Conjugated antisynovium when preceded only by normal rabbit immunoglobulin stained all the tissues examined except the glomerulus (lines 1 and 3). Pretreatment with unlabeled antiglomerulus abolished all staining by labeled antisynovium (lines 2 and 4), but pretreatment with unlabeled antisynovium did not abolish the staining of the glomerular basement membrane by labeled antiglomerulus (lines 6 and 8). This shows that the glomerulus contains a specific antigen plus an antigen that evokes antibodies cross-reactive with the other tissues under examination. The synovium, on the other hand, contains an antigen that evokes antibodies cross-reactive with peritubular capillaries, vascular adventitia, and splenic reticulum, but not with the second antigen in the glomerular basement membrane. The orange-red glomerular fluorescence due to RH-antiglomerulus was not altered by even prolonged treatment with FITC-antisynovium (line 11), nor was the green fluorescence of FITC-antiglomerulus affected by treatment with RH-antisynovium (line 14). However, short treatment with FITC-antisynovium altered the rhodamine fluorescence from antiglomerulus in the vascular adventitia (line 9), while more prolonged treatment was necessary to alter the color in the peritubular capillaries, the reticulum, and the synovium (lines 10 and 11). Consonant results were obtained with RH-antisynovium followed by FITC anti-glomerulus (lines 12 to 14). This shows that antisynovium reacts much stronger than antiglomerulus with the vascular adventitia, or that the cross-reactions

Table 2-2

Antibody exchange on sequential application to cross-reacting antigens, double-staining technique

Line no.	First treatment of section *	Second treatment of section	Hours of Second treatment	Kidney			Spleen	Synovium
				Glomerular membrane	Peritubular capillaries	Vascular adventitia	Reticulum	Cells
1	NRG	F antisyn	½-¾	—	G	G	G	G
2	antiglom	F antisyn	½-¾	—	—	—	—	—
3	NRG	R antisyn	½-¾	—	OR	OR	OR	OR
4	antiglom	R antisyn	½-¾	—	—	—	—	—
5	NRG	F antiglom	½-¾	G	G	G	G	G
6	antisyn	F antiglom	½-¾	G	—	—	—	—
7	NRG	R antiglom	½-¾	OR	OR	OR	OR	OR
8	antisyn	R antiglom	½-¾	OR	—	—	—	—
9	R antiglom	F antisyn	½	OR	OR	YO	OR	OR
10	R antiglom	F antisyn	2	OR	OY	G	OY	YO
11	R antiglom	F antisyn	18	OR	Y	G	Y	Y
12	F antiglom	R antisyn	¾	G	G	G	G	G
13	F antiglom	R antisyn	3	G	GY	OY	GY	GY
14	F antiglom	R antisyn	18	G	Y	O	Y	Y
15	R antisyn	F antiglom	½	G	O	OR	O	O
16	R antisyn	F antiglom	2	G	Y	O	YO	YO
17	R antisyn	F antiglom	18	G	G	O	GY	GY
18	F antisyn	R antiglom	¾	OR	G	O	G	G
19	F antisyn	R antiglom	3	OR	Y	G	YO	Y
20	F antisyn	R antiglom	18	OR	Y	G	YO	YO

Application of conjugated immunoglobulin to varying tissues delineates its extent of reactivity. Sequential application of unlabeled followed by homologous or cross-reacting immunoglobulin delineates their specificities. Sequential application of FITC (respectively RH)—labeled immunoglobulin and RH (respectively FITC)—labeled immunoglobulin delineates cross-reactivity by color of fluorescence emission. Adapted from D. C. Scott, *Immunology*, 3:226, 1960. F: Fluorescein conjugate; R: Lissamine rhodamine B200 conjugate; antiglom: antiglomerulus globulin; antisyn: antisynovium globulin; OR: orange-red color; O: orange; OY: orange predominates over yellow; YO: yellow predominates over orange; G: green; GY: green predominates over yellow; Y: yellow.

* The first treatment was for 18 hours.

52

of the antibodies to the second (cross-reactive) glomerular antigen with the vascular adventitia are weaker than with the other antigens. Consonant results were also obtained in the reverse situation when FITC (respectively RH)-conjugated antiglomerulus followed treatment with RH (respectively FITC)-antisynovium. Now prolonged treatment by the second conjugate was required to obtain fluorescence color change, if any, in the adventitia (lines 16, 17, 19, and 20), while treatment for ½ to 3 hours led to mixed color fluorescence in the peritubular capillaries, the reticulum, and the synovium (lines 15 and 19). It can be concluded without even producing an antiserum to splenic reticulum that reticulum and certain connective tissue fibrils are antigenically dissimilar.

CONTROLS

Satisfactory controls require that the microscopic field looks dark except for the faint bluish autofluorescence of tissues.

The *staining controls* are as follows:

1. Exposure to all staining reagents of tissue from the same host known not to contain the antigen under investigation.

2. In the direct method, preabsorption of the conjugate with the tissue under investigation.

3. In the indirect method, preabsorption of the unlabeled specific antiserum with the tissue under examination.

4. In the indirect method, omission of the unlabeled specific antiserum.

5. In the direct method, blocking of the reaction with the conjugate by pretreatment with unconjugated serum. The control depends on the fast reaction of antigen with antibody and the relatively slow reverse reaction in most systems. The blocking reaction is favored by low temperature, low concentration of the conjugate, and short exposure time to the conjugate. The inhibition is more likely to be successful if the conjugate is of poor quality, that is of low antibody content. Consequently, a not entirely satisfactory blocking control does not necessarily indicate nonspecificity.

6. In the indirect method, blocking the fluorescence by staining with specific antiserum followed by unlabeled anti-IgG and then labeled anti-IgG.

The *antibody controls* are as follows:

1. In the direct method, exposure of the tissue to conjugated normal immunoglobulin or immunoglobulin of unrelated specificities.

2. In the indirect method, substitution of the unlabeled antiserum by normal serum or antiserum of unrelated specificity.

3. In the direct method, absorption of the conjugate with the specific antigen under investigation.

4. In the indirect method, absorption of the unlabeled antiserum with the specific antigen under investigaition.

5. Evaluation of the cross-reactivity of two antisera as described on page 51 and in Table 2-2.

APPLICATIONS

Immunofluorescence has advanced many areas of biologic research; it has been essential to some. Autoimmunity as a factor in many chronic diseases of previously unknown etiology has been the direct result of immunofluorescence research. New insight into the causation of cancer under the concept of neoplastic transformation has been possible by research in immunofluorescence. Since immunologists developed immunofluorescence, it is natural that Coons and his students applied the technique in its very early stages to the study of antibody formation. Separate chapters will be devoted to some applications of immunocytochemistry that are largely due to immunofluorescence (Chapters 8 and 9). The bulk of the remaining applications cannot be dealt with here. Diagnostic immunofluorescence includes, for example, methods of typing cultured bacteria, identifying bacteria in tissue sections of autopsy material without recourse to culture, detection of antibodies against organisms that cannot be cultured (such as treponemal immunofluorescence with syphilitic serum), diagnosis of malaria, amebiasis, schistosomiasis, trichinosis, visceral leishmaniasis, and trypanosomiasis, identification of influenza virus in sputum smears, and typing of adenoviruses.

Rarely has a single technique had as profound an impact to progress of science as immunofluorescence. It is, perhaps, the wealth of application rather than shortcomings of techique that has prompted the search for even better methods of immunocytochemistry. The restriction of immunofluorescence to light microscopic resolutions has prompted, of course, the search for methods for electron microscopic immunocytochemistry. The high sensitivity of immunofluorescence despite losses of antibody activity during conjugation has prompted the search for methods that are even more sensitive. In the discourse that follows, we will learn initially about methods that increase the resolution from light to electron microscopy and later about methods that increase sensitivity in both light and electron microscopy.

REFERENCES

Arnold, W. and Von Mayersbach, H. Changes in solubility of immunoglobulins after fluorescent labeling and its influences on immunofluorescent technics. *J. Histochem. Cytochem.,* **20**:975, 1972.

Beutner, E., ed. Defined immunofluorescent staining. *Annals N.Y. Acad. Med.,* **177**, 1971.

Coons, A. H. and Kaplan, M. H. Localization of antigens in tissue cells. II. Improvement in a method for the detection of antigen by means of fluorescent antibody. *J. Exp. Med.,* **91**:1, 1950.

Engelhardt, N. V., Gousser, A. I., Shipora, L. J., and Abeler, G. I. Immunofluorescent study of alpha-fetoprotein (αfp) in liver and liver tumours. I. Technique of αfp localization in tissue sections. *Int. J. Cancer,* **7**:198, 1971.

Hardy, P. H. and Nell, E. E. Characteristics of fluorescein labeled antiglobulin preparations that may affect the fluorescent treponemal antibody-absorption test. *Am. J. Clin. Path.,* **56**:181, 1971.

Morikawa, S., Yamamura, M., Harada, T., and Hamashima, Y. Studies on cross-reactivity of antiribonuclease antisera with heterologous mammalian ribonucleotides. *J. Histochem. Cytochem.,* **16**:410, 1968.

Nairn, R. C., ed. *Fluorescent Protein Tracing* (3rd ed.) E. N. S. Livingstone, Ltd., Edinburgh and London. 1969.

Nash, D. R., Crabbé, P. A., and Heremans, J. F. Sequential immunofluorescent staining: a simple and useful technique. *Immunology,* **16**:785, 1969.

Pollak, V. E., Ooi, B. S., and Pesce, A. J. The distribution of serum albumin in the diseased human nephron as determined by immunofluorescense. *J. Lab. Clin. Med.,* **76**:357, 1970.

Schechter, I. Mapping of the combining sites of antibodies specific for poly-L-alanine determinants. *Nature,* **228**:639, 1970.

Scott, D. G. Immunohistochemical studies of connective tissue: The use of contrasting fluorescent protein tracers in the comparison of two antisera. *Immunology,* **3**:226, 1960.

Von Mayersbach, H., ed. Immunohistochemistry. *Acta, Histochemica,* Suppl. 7, Gustav Fischer Verlag. Jena, 1967.

Von Mayersbach, H. Immunohistology. In *Handbook of Histochemistry,* Vol. 1, General Methodology, 2nd part (Grauman, W. and Neumann, K. eds.) Gustav Fischer Verlag. Stuttgart, 1966.

Chapter 3

The Immunoferritin Method

We have seen in the preceding chapter that the labeling of an antibody molecule with strongly absorbing dye molecules does not yield enough color contrast for visualization of antigen by light microscopy. For similar reasons the labeling of an antibody molecule with one to three atoms of a metal, even a high atomic number metal, does not yield enough electron opacity for visualization of antigen on the photgraphic plate of the electron microscope. We have seen that in light microscopy the problem was solved by substituting for light absorption against a bright background secondary light emission against a dark background in the form of fluorescence. For electron microscopic immunocytochemistry an approach must be used that is analogous to the insensitive, dye-conjugated, light absorbing antibodies in light microscopy. Successful electron microscopy by this approach requires that the number of electron-opaque atoms per molecule of antibody is increased far beyond the number of fluorescent groups per molecule of antibody needed for light microscopy. To make this possible new procedures had to be developed that bear little resemblance to conjugation of one molecule of fluorescent dye to one molecule of antibody. Many of these new procedures brought new problems as well. These problems laid heavily on the progress of immune electron microscopy in its infancy. Their solutions have required fundamental departures from the methods originally introduced.

Electron opacity can be conferred to the site of an antigen-antibody reaction by *directly labeling* the antibody with a heavy metal, by attaching to the antibody by covalent or immunologic bonds a molecule that possesses characteristically *structured electron opacity,* or by bringing specifically to the site of the antigen-antibody reaction an *enzyme* that can be detected by formation of an opaque product.

Direct labeling

Iodine, diazotized tetraacetoxymercuric salicylate, or p-aminophenyl mercuric acetate, or ferrocene (*bis*-pentadienyl iron) fail to confer suffi-

56

cient electron opacity to antibody because it is necessary to restrict the number of labeling groups per antibody moleclue. Antibody reactivity becomes reduced to approximately ½ when about ten labeling residues have reacted per antibody molecule. Little antibody activity remains when 30 residues have reacted. Ten mercury atoms increase the density of antibody by 1.3% and 30 atoms by 4%, which is insufficient for detection in the electron microscope. A more satisfactory extent of conjugation of antibodies with metal can be achieved if the antibody combining sites are specifically protected during conjugation. Reaction with antigen affords such protection. The label will react with available sites on the antibody molecule to the exclusion of the specific combining regions that are occupied by antigen. The procedure is conveniently combined with preparation of purified antibody. Antibody is removed from serum by a specific immunoabsorbent. While the antibody is on the immunoabsorbent, an exhaustive amount of uranyl acetate is applied to chelate extensively with the antibody, and the purified, labeled antibody is eluted from the immunoabsorbent by brief treatment with cold alkali. The antibody contains 200 atoms of uranium per molecule while retaining its specific reactivity with antigen. Density is increased by 40%. This extent of contrast is sufficient for electron microscopy when the concentration of antigen is high within a surrounding tissue that is not itself counterstained or fixed with electron-opaque fixative, such as osmium tetroxide. After completion of the immunologic reaction with uranium-labeled antibody on the thin section of the electron microscopy specimen, the specific contrast of the antibody can be enhanced by ligating one arm of thiocarbohydrazide, a double-armed hydrazine ligand, onto the bound uranium in the antibody and then chelating osmium tetroxide onto the remaining free hydrazine arm. The density of antibody thus increases by 65–190%, depending upon the number of osmium atoms bridged to each uranium atom via thiocarbohydrazide. Although this method of conferring electron opacity onto antibody proves to be of satisfactory specificity, the degree of attainable opacity still restricts it to antigens of high concentration, such as viruses or lysosomal enzymes, at relatively low magnification. The method becomes insensitive at low concentrations of antigens and at high magnification.

An explanation for the loss of differential contrast of uranium-labeled antibody with surrounding structure at high resolution has been provided by H. Tanaka. In order to give distinct contrast with surrounding areas, the value of $NZ^{4/3}/S$ for a specifically stained area should be greater than $4700/nm^2$, where N is the number of heavy metal atoms of atomic number Z added as a label to an area of size S. If we assume the area of a single antibody molecule to be 76 nm^2, the value of $NZ^{4/3}/S$ is $45/nm^2$ for a molecule of antibody labeled with 10 mercury atoms, $134/nm^2$ for a molecule labeled with 30 mercury atoms, $944/nm^2$ if labeled with 200 uranium

atoms, and 1935/nm^2 if the uranium is bridged to osmium via thiocarbohydrazide at a ratio of one osmium to one uranium atom. Even the value
for osmium-bridged uranium antibody is too low for distinction of single
molecules at high resolution. Useful contrast can only be obtained at lower
resolution when the concentration of antigen is high, especially upon application of antibody to the thin section of the electron microscopy specimen
by the indirect method in which several antibody molecules are packed on
top of each other, thus increasing N in $NZ^{4/3}/S$.

Structured electron opacity

Ferritin has been introduced by Singer and Schick as a marker that possesses characteristic structured electron opacity. Ferritin is a spherical molecule with a diameter of 12 nm, a molecular weight of 650,000, and an iron

Fig. 3-1 Sheep red cells (SRBC) reacted with ferritin-conjugated immunoglobulin anti-SRBC
diluted 1:10 (agglutinin titer was 1:40). Individual ferritin molecules can always be discerned
in the immunoferritin method because the iron micelles in the core of the molecule are surrounded by the electron-translucent sheet of the bulk of the ferritin molecule. Although the
distribution of antigen on the erythrocyte membrane is continuous (page 173), localization of
ferritin appears in clusters suggesting that the localized material does not only consist of
monomeric, but also of polymeric aggregates of ferritin with immunoglobulin. Arrow shows intercellular immunoglobulin bridge. From H. Schäfer, *Immunoelectron microscopy*, Gustav Fischer
Verlag, Stuttgart, 1971.

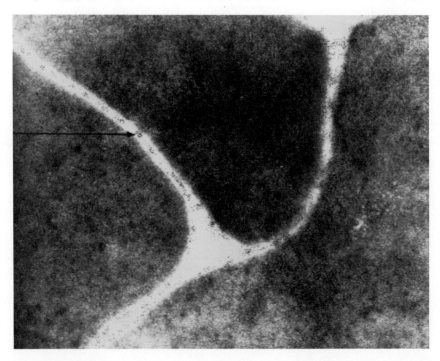

content of 23% by weight. Were the iron distributed uniformly the electron contrast, $NZ^{4/5}/S$, would only be $1030/nm^2$, and single molecules could not be distinguished from surrounding structures. Fortunately, the iron is concentrated in characteristic micelles in the center of the molecule forming a tetrad with a diameter of 5 nm. This affords a high concentration of iron and characteristic structure at single molecule resolution. $NZ^{4/3}/S$ for the tetrad is $6000/nm$, well above the value needed for good differential contrast. When ferritin is conjugated to antibody covalently, the point of electron opacity is seen at a distance of about 8 nm from the point of attachment of the ferritin with the antibody (Fig. 3–1).

Enzymes

Enzymes can be used in immunoelectron microscopy either covalently conjugated with antibody (Chapter 5) or attached to the site of the antigen-antibody reaction in the specimen via unlabeled antibodies only (Chapter 6). Depending upon their manner of use, enzymes can afford an amplification over the specific contrast attainable with other methods.

CONJUGATION OF FERRITIN WITH IMMUNOGLOBULIN: PRINCIPLE

For the covalent binding of ferritin with immunoglobulin, a bifunctional or double-armed reagent is needed: one arm for conjugation with ferritin and the other for conjugation with immunoglobulin. If both proteins and a bifunctional reagent are mixed, it is difficult to control the fast reaction of the relatively small molecular double-armed reagent with one of the macromolecular proteins and the succeeding, but slower reaction of a conjugated with an unconjugated macromolecular protein. An excess of bifunctional reagent would be needed to drive the slower reaction. Such excess of bifunctional reagent would cause extensive destruction of antibody activity and would lead to uncontrollable amounts of polymeric aggregates of ferritin with immunoglobulin, or of immunoglobulin with immunoglobulin, or of ferritin with ferritin.

Conjugation in two stages and use of toluene-2,4-diisocyanate as conjugating reagent avoids most of these difficulties (Fig. 3–2).

In the *first* stage ferritin only is reacted with an excess of toluene diisocyanate at pH 7.5. Two factors insure that for the most part only one of the isocyanate groups reacts with a ferritin molecule, while the other group remains free. First, in toluene diisocyanate both isocyanate groups do not possess equal reactivity. The group in position 2 is partially hindered by the adjacent methyl group, so that under conditions of excess of reagent the

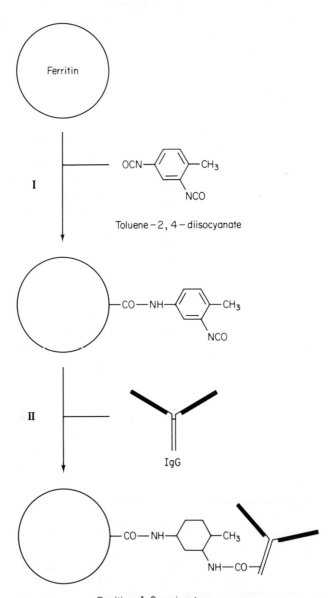

Fig. 3-2 Conjugation of ferritin with 2,4-toluene diisocyanate. In the first stage a number of toluene diisocyanate molecules reacts with each ferritin molecule, forming carbamido bonds between the 4-isocyanate groups and the free amino groups in ferritin. In the second stage the conjugated ferritin reacts with immunoglobulin forming carbamido bonds between the 2-isocyanate groups and the free amino groups of immunoglobulin. Limitation of reaction in the first stage insures that most reacting components in the second stage yield only dimers.

isocyanate in position *4* reacts preferentially. Second, pH 7.5 is below the optimum pH for reaction of isocyanate with amine, again disfavoring reaction of the 2-isocyanate and further mitigating against hydrolysis of the 2-isocyanate to the amine prior to separation of the reacted ferritin with unreacted excess of conjugant in preparation for the second step. As the immunoferritin method utilizes only the structural features of iron in ferritin rather than any special function of ferritin, it is not essential to avoid alteration of the ferritin molecule caused by excess of bifunctional reagent. Nevertheless, some of the difficulties in the more critical use of the immunoferritin method may in part be due to excessive amounts of toluene amine (hydrolyzed isocyanate) attached to the ferritin surface.

In the *second* stage the diisocyanate-reacted ferritin is admixed with immunoglobulin at pH 9.5. The immunoglobulin never encounters any unreacted *di*isocyanate and, hence, destruction of antibody activity is minimized. At pH 9.5 the isocyanate group in the 2-position becomes reactive with antibody amine; yet the alkalinity is not so high as to irreversibly destroy antibody activity. Ferritin now can only react with immunoglobulin. Side reactions of immunoglobulin with immunoglobulin are avoided because

Fig. 3-3 Products of reaction of limited conjugation of ferritin with specific immunoglobulin followed by purification of conjugates. *a* and *b* are specifically reacting constituents of the conjugate. *c* and *d* do not react specifically and may contribute to nonspecific staining. Nonspecific immunoglobulin is marked by X at the N-terminal portion of the Fab fragments (page 6). Fe, ferritin.

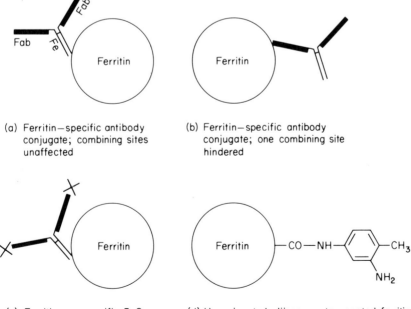

(a) Ferritin–specific antibody conjugate; combining sites unaffected

(b) Ferritin–specific antibody conjugate; one combining site hindered

(c) Ferritin–nonspecific IgG conjugate

(d) Unconjugated, diisocyanate–reacted ferritin (only one of many reacted diisocyanate groups is shown) of the absence of free diisocyanate, and side reactions of ferritin with ferritin are avoided because the ferritin already has been reacted exhaustively with diisocyanate. Hence, the first reaction step that occurs in the second stage is always formation of the desired dimer consisting of one ferritin and one immunoglobulin molecule irrespective of the proportion of ferritin and immunoglobulin monomeres in the mixture (Fig. 3–3). If the reaction is allowed to proceed, the dimer will react either with another immunoglobulin molecule, or with another ferritin molecule, or with another dimer (Fig. 3–4). Eventually, this continued polymerization becomes restricted by hydrolysis of the 2-isocyanate on the reactive ferritin.

When one ferritin molecule has reacted with one immunoglobulin molecule, only one and never both of the antibody combining sites can be affected by steric hindrance. At worst, antibody would become monovalent (unable to precipitate with antigen), but in any event would still be able to combine with antigen and, hence, would still be useful for immunocytochemical localization. In fact, even hindrance of one specific combining site in an immunoglobulin molecule is not necessarily the rule upon reaction with a single ferritin molecule. However, if the reaction is permitted to proceed to large aggregates, steric hindrance becomes likely both by conjugation onto additional ferritin molecules or ferritin-immunoglobulin complexes. Since in IgG preparations only a relatively small proportion of molecules are specific antibody, chances are high that polymerization with additional IgG will only add bulk but not specific reactivity to a specific antibody-ferritin conjugate.

For these reasons it is important to limit the extent of reaction in the second stage to a yield of 20–30% in conjugate. Under such limitation the bulk of immunoglobulin and ferritin remain unconjugated.

The reaction in the second stage is not easily terminated. Instead, limitation of the second stage is done by limiting the time and, hence, the extent of reaction of ferritin with 2,4-toluene diisocyanate in the first stage.

In contrast to toluene diisocyanate, bifunctional reagents in which both groups are of equal reactivity, like xylylene diisocyanate, glutaraldehyde, or difluorodinitrodiphenyl sulphone (FNPS) must be employed in large excess in the first stage to insure that unreacted ferritin-bound isocyanate groups are available for the second stage. Hence, these reagents are not suitable for limiting the reaction in the second stage to formation of dimeric conjugate. At times it is even necessary to use glutaraldehyde or FNPS in a single stage procedure, thus, losing all the advantages of sequential conjugation.

Unconjugated antibodies block the reaction of tissue antigen with ferritin-conjugated antibodies. The weight differential of conjugated and unconjugated antibodies permits their separation. However, S. Marinis and A. Vogt have shown that high speed-centrifuged conjugate retains nearly

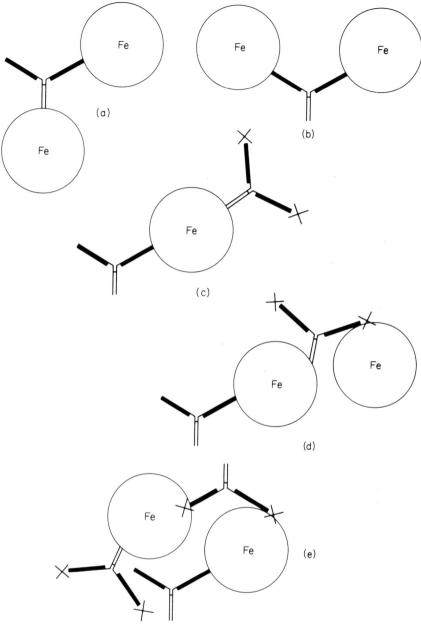

Fig. 3-4 Some products of conjugation of ferritin and immunoglobulin resulting in addition to those shown in Fig. 3-3 upon extensive (high yield) conjugation of ferritin with immunoglobulin. (a). 2 ferritin-1 specific antibody, specifically active conjugate. (b). 2 ferritin-1 specific antibody, sterically hindered conjugate, (c). 1 ferritin-1 specific antibody-1 nonspecific IgG, specifically active conjugate. (d). 2 ferritin-1 specific antibody—1 nonspecific IgG, specifically active conjugate. (e). 2 ferritin-1 specific antibody—2 nonspecific IgG. One antibody site is sterically hindered by conjugation with one ferritin and the other by the bulk of surrounding ferritin and nonspecific IgG. Large complexes are undesirable because of increased tendency to nonspecific adherence to tissue.

63

50% of the contaminating, unconjugated globulin (Fig. 3–5). Hence, it is desirable to recentrifuge the pellet, preferably on a sucrose density gradient, to determine both ferritin and protein contents of each collected fraction and to use only those fractions that are free of unconjugated immunoglobulin. These fractions still contain unconjugated ferritin. Alternatively, the redissolved pellet can be separated by zonal electrophoresis into the slowly migrating unconjugated IgG, the fast migrating unconjugated ferritin and the conjugate of intermediate mobility. Success of this separation depends upon using IgG_2 for conjugation, because other immunoglobulin classes overlap in mobility with ferritin-IgG_2 conjugate.

Fig. 3-5 Sucrose density gradients of the products of limited conjugation of ferritin with ^{125}I-IgG partially purified by a single sedimentation at 40,000 rpm for one hour (Spinco rotor 40). Radioactivity in counts per minute ($\times$); ferritin concentration in OD at 440 nm (o). Concentration of IgG in OD at 280 nm (o). Counts and OD_{440} are parallel until the peak tube (fraction 40). Heavy contamination of unconjugated immunoglobulin peaks near fraction 60. Lack of parallelism of counts and OD_{440} between tubes 40 and 50 indicates contamination by unconjugated immunoglobulin. To obtain ferritin-immunoglobulin conjugates free of nonspecific immunoglobulin, only the OD_{440} peak tube and heavier fractions should be pooled. From S. Marinis, A. Vogt, and G. Brandner, *Immunology*, **17**:77, 1969.

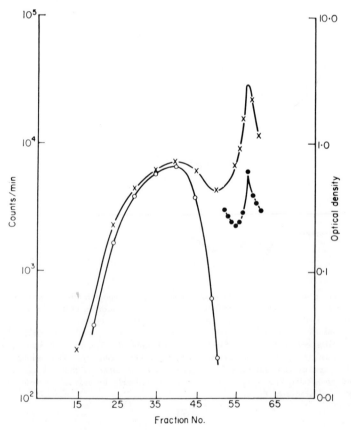

Measurement of antibody activity in conjugates by tests that depend on precipitation, agglutination, or other secondary phenomena in the antigen antibody reaction may give erroneously high or low estimates. Ferritin, especially isocyanate-conjugated ferritin, possesses a tendency to adsorb nonspecifically on surfaces. This tendency may increase nonspecifically the amount of precipitate obtained upon reaction of conjugate with specific antigen. On the other hand, steric hindrance of one of the combining sites of IgG by conjugation with ferritin would result in monovalent antibody that would not only fail to precipitate with antigen but also interfere with the precipitation of divalent antibody and antigen. In general, if the conjugation reaction is not limited to below 30% yield, specific precipitation or agglutination of isolated conjugate (free of unconjugated antibody) is entirely abolished or severely reduced.

The unreliability of agglutination for estimating retention of antibody activity upon conjugation can be illustrated by the localization of specific conjugate on the sheep erythrocyte (SRBC) surface in the studies of H. Schäfer (Fig. 3-1). Xylylene diisocyanate-prepared conjugate was found after three high speed centrifugations to be electrophoretically free of unconjugated immunoglobulin. The localization of conjugate was patchy even though used at a concentration four times in excess of that required for cell agglutination. In contrast, unlabeled antibody gives patchy localization only when diluted to its agglutination titer or beyond (analyzed by a different immunocytochemical method, page 173). Apparently, conjugation enhances agglutination by nonspecific forces.

This illustrates the need for a primary binding test of antibody activity in conjugate. A mixture of antihuman serum albumin (anti-HSA) and a fair excess of ^{131}I-HSA separates on electrophoresis into a fast moving component of free antigen, a slower moving component consisting of complexes of excess antigen with antibody, and a component of precipitated, or at least polymerized antigen-antibody complexes that stays at the origin (Fig. 3-6). When ferritin-conjugated immunoglobulin is prepared from ^{125}I-immunoglobulin anti-HSA under conditions of limited conjugation, a fixed amount of ^{131}I-HSA admixed with equal numbers of ^{125}I counts of conjugated or unconjugated immunoglobulin gives identical electrophorograms, showing that essentially all specific binding activity of the antibody in the conjugate is retained.

Identical specific binding activity for sheep erythrocytes (SRBC) was found by Fresen and Vogt for radioiodinated, unconjugated immunoglobulin anti-SRBC and its ferritin-conjugates prepared and purified on sucrose density gradients. Hemoagglutination that requires more than one intact antibody combining site is severely reduced or entirely abolished in such conjugates. Interestingly, hemolytic activity with complement is reduced 16-fold. Hemolysis by IgG and complement occurs only if at least

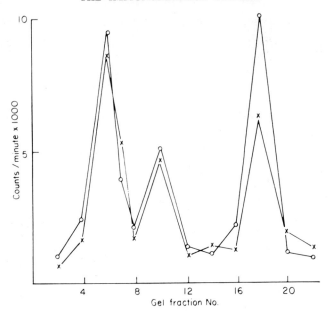

Fig. 3-6 Distribution of ^{131}I radioactivity on electrophoretic separation in acrylamide gel of mixtures of ^{131}I-human serum albumin (HSA) with ^{125}I-IgG anti-HSA (✗) and with an equal amount of ^{125}I counts of ferritin-conjugated ^{125}I-IgG anti-HSA (o). The conjugate was prepared under conditions of limited yield, purified by high speed centrifugation and zonal gradient sedimentation. Identity of both electrophorograms attest to retention of antibody activity in the conjugate. From Ursula Birnbaum, A. Vogt, and S. Marinis, *Immunology*, **18**:443, 1970.

two IgG molecules are bound to the cell in immediate juxtaposition. Apparently, the conjugation with ferritin prevents this juxtaposition.

Vogt has shown that unconjugated ferritin or nonspecific conjugate are rapidly cleared from the kidney of rats one day after injection. Similarly, rabbit immunoglobulin antirat kidney extensively conjugated with ferritin fails to be retained in rat kidneys more than one day after injection. Hence, no injected ferritin or conjugate is expected to be localized nonspecifically beyond one day after injection. Conjugate prepared under yield limitation below 30% localizes specifically and uniformly on the endothelial side of the basement membrane and remains attached with a half-life of 6–18 days (Fig. 3-7). Specific localization with carefully prepared conjugate contrasts with the entire lack of specificity of conjugate prepared under less exacting conditions. The finding serves to illustrate the importance of limited extent of conjugation followed by monitored separation of unconjugated antibody. Even though these precautions complicate somewhat the technique of conjugation and decrease the yield, they seem to be essential for the more exacting requirements of electron microscopic resolution compared to those of light microscopy.

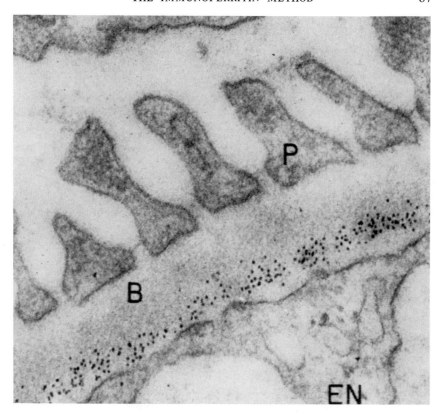

Fig. 3-7 Part of a glomerulus from a rat receiving 12 mg of rabbit serum antirat kidney conjugated with ferritin, examined three days after injection. Any nonspecifically localized material had cleared the kidney after the first day. The conjugate prepared under mild conditions (limited yield) deposits uniformly on the endothelial side of the basement membrane (B). This contrasts with a more patchy deposition on the cell surface *in vitro* of more extensively reacted conjugate in Fig. 3-1. The endothelial cell (EN) appears to be swollen and is partially separated from the basement membrane. Epithelial foot processes (P) are not altered. X117,000. From A. Vogt, H. Bockhorn, K. Kozina, and M. Sasaki, *J. Exp. Med.* **128:867,** 1968.

Conjugation of Ferritin with Immunoglobulin: Techniques

Commercial ferritin preparations are often contaminated with large amounts of apoferritin (ferritin devoid of heme) that must be removed to avoid formation of conjugates that competively block reaction of ferritin-conjugated antibody. Make up 1 gm of crude ferritin (twice crystallized and once precipitated) to 100 ml with a 2% solution of ammonium sulfate. Add 33.3 ml of a 20% solution of cadmium sulfate. Allow to crystallize at 1–6° for one day. Centrifuge and dissolve precipitate in 100 ml of the 2%

ammonium sulfate solution. Recentrifuge, collect supernate, and add 33.3 ml of a 20% solution of cadmium sulfate. Again allow to crystallize at 1–6° for one day. If the suspension contains noncrystallized material in addition to the crystals, repeat the procedure until the suspension in cadmium sulfate is free of noncrystallized material. Centrifuge and dissolve precipitate in 75 ml of the 2% ammonium sulfate solution. Add 75 ml of a saturated solution of ammonium sulfate, allow to stand for one hour at 1–6°, centrifuge and dissolve precipitate in 75 ml of water. Reprecipitate in ammonium sulfate twice, suspend in a small volume of water, dialyze against running tap water in the cold overnight and then against 0.05 M phosphate buffer, pH 7.5. Centrifuge dialysate at 35,000 rpm for two hours (Spinco Rotor 40). Remove the colorless top portion of the solution. Dissolve the pellet in the dark bottom portion of the solution. Either use the solution immediately or centrifuge at 4,000 rpm (Sorvall Rotor SM24) for 30 minutes at 1–6° and sterilize by passage through a Millipore filter. Store solution at 1–6°. Determine protein contents of the ferritin solution.

The *conjugation of ferritin with immunoglobulin* is done between 0 and 5°. Make up 150 mg of ferritin to 6.0 ml with phosphate buffer, pH 7.5, 0.05 M in phosphate, 0.15 M in sodium chloride. Add under stirring 0.15 ml of 2,4-toluene diisocyanate. Continue stirring for 20 minutes while maintaining pH at 7.5 with sodium carbonate solution. Centrifuge at 15,000 rpm for five minutes (Sorvall Rotor SM24). Pipette the clear supernatant into a graduated container, record volume, and let stand for 10 minutes to minimize any residual, unreacted diisocyanate.

For *stage two* admix a volume of the supernate containing 125 mg ferritin with an equal volume of immunoglobulin containing 125 mg protein and an equal volume of 0.3 M sodium carbonate buffer, pH 9.5. Stir mixture for 48 hours. Dialyze against 15 liters of 0.1 M ammonium carbonate solution and then against 15 liters of phosphate buffer, pH 7.5, 0.05 M in phosphate, 0.15 M in sodium chloride. Centrifuge at 15,000 rpm at 1–6° for 5 minutes.

For purification of the conjugate (following the procedure of Marinis) place supernate into Spinco tubes containing about 1 ml of a thick suspension of Sephadex G25 and centrifuge at 40,000 rpm for one hour (Spinco Rotor 40). Dissolve sediment in a small volume of phosphate buffer (the Sephadex aids solution of the pellet). If it is desirable to remove all unconjugated antibody, place solution on a discontinuous sucrose gradient (60, 45, and 30%) and centrifuge at 25,600 rpm for 4–5 hours (Spinco Rotor SW25). Record OD_{440} and OD_{280} of each fraction and collect the peak fraction as measured by absorbence at 440 nm and the fractions heavier than the peak fraction. Discard the fractions lighter than the peak fraction. Discard a pellet if it forms. Dialyze against phosphate buffer pH 7.5, 0.05

M in phosphate, 0.15 M in sodium chloride, and concentrate on an Amicon membrane. Pass solution through a sterile Millipore filter and keep at 1–6°.

STAINING

For application of antibodies, similar principles prevail as in immuno-fluorescence. Direct and indirect techniques are used (page 36), and the necessary controls are analogous (page 53). For localization of antigen on the surface of cells, it is often of value to keep them alive at least during the first application of antibody. Problems arise in the staining of the interior of the cell. We remember that in immunofluorescence the interior of the cell is made accessible by preparing sections 1–6 μ thick prior to staining, thereby cutting the cells open. The resolution of electron microscopy requires, however, that not only the cell but also subcellular organelles, membranes, and channels are cut open by microtomy. Antibodies do not penetrate subcellular membranes just as they fail to penetrate the outer cell or plasma membrane. To assure accessibility, the microtomy section should be of sufficient thinness (30–100 nm), and the staining with conjugate should be done on such sections. Fixation of tissue, dehydration, and embedding in plastic are necessary in order to confer upon the tissue the necessary mechanical stability for ultrathin sectioning. Antigen reactivity must be maintained in this procedure. Also, accessibility of antigen embedded in plastic to antibodies applied to the ultrathin section must be assured. Although staining on the section is possible, at least for some antigens, in three different methods of electron microscopic immunocytochemistry, staining on the section with ferritin-labeled antibodies has largely been nonspecific. The nonspecificity is due to binding of ferritin-labeled antibodies or of ferritin itself with the plastic embedding medium, thereby over-shadowing any specific localization in the tissue itself. This nonspecificity cannot be overcome by substitution of the common embedding media with media made from hydrophilic or charged monomers. Consequently, staining by the immunoferritin method must be done prior to embedding. The cell as well as membranes in the interior of the cells must be made accessible to antibodies. Fixation in itself as it affects the living membrane potential aids penetration of antibodies. Freezing and thawing increase penetrability further as formation of ice crystals traumatizes the membranes. The procedure affects ultrastructure severely, but prior fixation may minimize the damage. Penetrability is also increased by use of digitonin or by dimethyl-sulfoxide. Damage to ultrastructure upon freezing may also be diminished if the temperature is lowered slowly and at a controlled rate, especially in the presence of 10% dimethylsulfoxide. G. Andres and his associates prefer freezing in 20% glycerol because of better structural preservation. The methods for promoting accessibility of antibodies to the interior of cells are usually less effective with solid tissues than with blood cells or tissue culture monolayer cells.

For the detection of many viral antigens, monolayer cells may be fixed in 4% formaldehyde in PBS for five minutes. Following three washings in PBS, the cells are treated with a 10% solution of dimethylsulfoxide in PBS for 30 minutes, then scraped off the flask, sedimented at low speed, quick frozen in dry ice, and thawed after three minutes.

In an application of this method by M. Wagner and A. Veckenstedt to the detection of mengovirus antigen 8–16 hours after infection of L-cells, the cells were exposed by the indirect method to guinea pig serum anti-mengo L-virus for one hour at 37°, washed twice with PBS for 10 minutes, incubated for one hour at 37° with ferritin-conjugated rabbit immunoglobulin antiguinea pig immunoglobulin and, again after thorough washing, fixed in buffered osmium tetroxide solution (1%), and embedded in Vestopal. Ferritin was localized in aggregates of unit size of 14 nm, probably circumscribing virus particles described as 16–28 nm in diameter. These viral aggregates were localized along a progressively developing system of cytoplasmic vesicles that form a flattened canalicular network and are probably the site of viral synthesis. The characteristic ferritin-localized particles were found in greatest frequency close to the cell membrane and at times apparently penetrating it. Viral protein unassociated with viral particles was seen as dispersed, cytoplasmic, ferritin-labeled granules.

Apparently the best cellular penetration, albeit with some sacrifice of specificity and antigenic reactivity, is accomplished by treatment with digitonin and fixation with glutaraldehyde. Cells are suspended in PBS containing 4×10^{-5} M digitonin and are fixed immediately in 1% glutaraldehyde for five minutes. Following centrifugation, pellets of cells cut into fragments (about 1 mm³) are washed with 3–4 changes of PBS over a period of 8–12 hours (Fig. 3–8).

A typical way of preparing and staining solid tissue has been described by G. Andres in a classical electron immunocytochemical contribution to immune complex disease (page 222). Renal biopsy material from patients with acute glomerulonephritis was fixed for one hour at 0° in 5% formalin in phosphate buffer, pH 7.2. The tissue was then cut in the cold into the smallest possible pieces obtainable under a dissecting microscope. The fragments were immersed in ferritin-conjugated immunoglobulin antihuman IgG, antihuman C3, or antistreptococcus type 12 for 20 minutes at room temperature, washed in phosphate buffer three times, fixed in 1% buffered osmium tetroxide, and embedded in Araldite. The simultaneous demonstration of human IgG, C3, and products of group A streptococci, and the

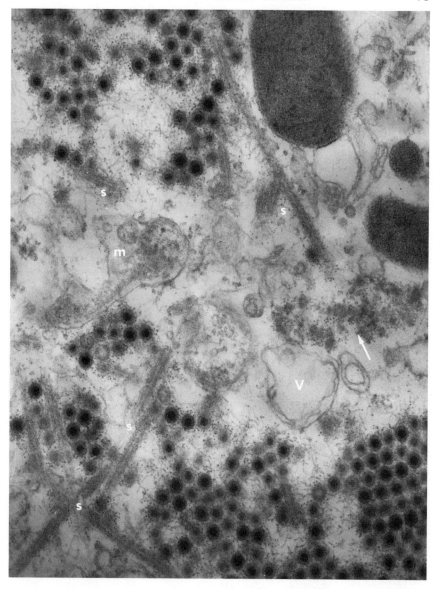

Fig. 3-8 L-cells treated with digitonin 12 hours after infection with reovirus. One-fourth to one-half of the cells treated had their outer cell membranes sufficiently disrupted to facilitate penetration of ferritin-labeled antibody. The interior of the cell also became more accessible to the label as evidenced from the specific tagging of viral particles in the exterior *as well as the interior* of the inclusion on top of the micrograph. Kinky filaments in proximity to the viral particles are devoid of ferritin. Specific label is also associated with the spindle tubules of the cell (s) and with amorphous material (arrows). m, mitochondria. V, vacuoles. From the work of S. Dales, P. J. Gomatos, and K. C. Hsu, *Virology,* **25**:193, 1965.

manner of their subcellular localization suggested that they represented antigen-antibody complexes caught in the filter system of the kidney.

APPLICATION: THE CELL SURFACE

The electron-lucent periphery of the ferritin molecule separates its electron-opaque core from adjacent molecules. Therefore, individual ferritin molecules can be distinguished and enumerated. If indeed a single ferritin molecule is conjugated to a single antibody molecule, then one ferritin core indicates localization of a single antibody molecule. Resolution of ultrastructure is only jeopardized to the extent that apposition of an antibody and a ferritin molecule enlarges the size of the structure observed.

On the human red cell surface the distribution of type A or Rh antigens was consistently found discontinuous: patchy clusters of ferritin are

Fig. 3-9 Localization of antigen sites on erythrocytes in two patients with autoimmune hemolytic anemia (a to c) [(a) and (b) from the same patient] and in a patient with penicillin-induced immune hemolytic anemia (d). The cells were incubated with ferritin-conjugated rabbit immunoglobulin anti-human IgG. X60,000. Distances (periodicities) of antigen sites (encircled) average 0.26 μ in (a), 0.42 μ in (b), 0.48 μ in (c), and 0.32 μ in (d). The individual aggregates of ferritin in (c) represent deposits of about 100 nm diameter, a very large aggregate for a single antigenic determinant on the cell. X60,000. From the work of W. C. Davis and co-workers, J. Immunol., 101:621, 1968.

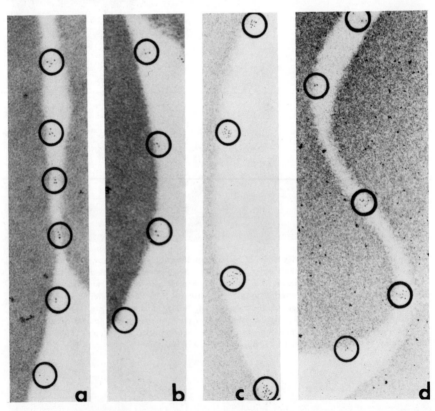

separated by stretches of cell surface devoid of ferritin. A similar distribution prevailed for receptors of myxoviruses that appear to be antigenically similar to blood group AB and O substances. Using the indirect technique, Davis and co-workers found in autoimmune hemolytic anemia periodicities of ferritin localization ranging from 0.21 to 0.46 μ in different patients [Fig. 3-9 (a), (b), and (c)] and in penicillin-induced hemolytic anemia a periodicity of 0.32 microns [Fig. 3-9 (d)]. In their study on RL antigen distribution, Davis and co-workers showed that the periodicity was not due to insufficient concentration of anti-RL sera or of the ferritin-labeled antiimmunoglobulin, since increase in concentration did not alter the pattern of localization. Increase in the ferritin-labeled antiimmunoglobulin did, however, increase the number of ferritin markers at any given site. If the assumption is made that a 1:1 ratio prevails between the number of ferritin *clusters* observed and the antigenic sites, a blood group O RL cell (genotype CDe/CDe) would possess 10,000 sites reacting with RL serum (anti-D). This corresponds well with the 15,000–19,000 sites determined wtih radioiodinated antiserum. However, the cells were unfixed, and the possibility of dislocation of antigen sites during staining must also be considered (page 103).

In the cascade of complement component activation by a single antigen-IgM antibody site on the red cell surface, components C1, C4, and C2 are activated in turn, and a single fragment of one molecule of each of these components is bound to one antigen-antibody site (EA) as EAC1a, 4,2a. It has been shown by radioiodinated antibody that each unit of such C1a,4,2a acts upon a large number of C3 molecules and converts them to an inactive form plus a lesser number of activated molecules that possess "stickiness" for certain receptor sites on the cell. Using a limited amount of antibody to sheep red cells and radioiodinated C4, Mardiney and co-workers localized EAC1,4,2a with ferritin-conjugated rabbit immunoglobulin anti-C4. The conjugated immunoglobulin had been effectively separated from unconjugated immunoglobulin, as well as from unconjugated ferritin by block electrophoresis. Localization of ferritin

Fig. 3-10 Sheep erythrocytes reacted with limited amounts of antibody and excess of complement components 1, 4, and 2. 450 molecules of radioiodinated component 4 have been bound. Upon incubation with ferritin-conjugated anti-C4, five deposits are seen as single or clustered ferritin granules. The deposits are widely separated in accordance with the small number of C4 molecules bound. X85,000. From M. R. Mardiney and co-workers, Am. J. Path., 53:253, 1968.

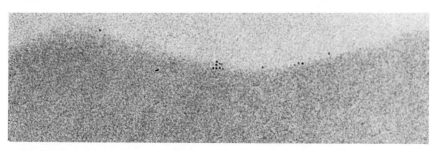

occurred in sparse clusters as expected (Fig. 3-10). An average of 1,400 ferritin molecules were counted per red cell. The number of C4 molecules as determined by bound radioactivity was 450. Hence, the average number of ferritin molecules per molecule of C4 was 3.1. Even though the localization of C4 was sparse, activated C3 was revealed either uniformly (Fig. 3-11) or in dense patches (Fig. 3-12) over the entire surface of the red cell, yielding an average of 100,000 ferritin particles per cell. With radioiodinated C3 the same number of molecules was found suggesting a 1:1 ratio of ferritin to C3. Interestingly, with this electrophoretically purified conjugate, the size of deposits, at least in some illustrations (Figs. 3-10 and 3-11) did not exceed 15 nm, suggesting a nonaggregated conjugate of single molecules of ferritin with single molecules of antibody. In the usual illustrations of surface antigen localized by ferritin-conjugated immunoglobulin, the maximum thickness of the deposit ranges from 60 nm in the direct to 100 nm in the indirect method, far exceeding the dimensions of a layer of unlabeled antibody plus a layer of conjugate of one ferritin with one immunoglobulin molecule.

The ferritin-conjugated antibody method has been useful in defining antigenic determinants on the surface of bacteria. Vegetative and spore forms of bacteria of the genus Bacillus as well as Clostridium present different antigens on their surfaces. In Clostridium, toxin production has long

Fig. 3-11 The red cell that has bound 450 molecules of C4 as EAC1a, 4, 2a complexes is reacted with C3 and ferritin-conjugated rabbit immunoglobulin anti-C3. In contrast to the sparse distribution of C4, C3 is attached over the entire cell surface. X95,000. From M. R. Mardiney and co-workers, Am. J. Path., 53:253, 1968.

Fig. 3-12 Sometimes in a preparation similar to that shown in Fig 3-11, C3 seems to be clustered. However, the number of the C3 sites still exceeds by far that of the C4 sites. In the clustered localization the width of the deposit exceeds that expected from the size of conjugate of a single ferritin with a single immunoglobulin molecule. X85,000. From M. R. Mardiney and co-workers, *Am. J. Path.*, **53**:253, 1968.

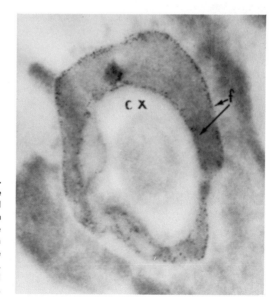

Fig. 3-13 A 20-hour culture of *C. botulinum* type A, unstabilized. The cell was treated with ferritin-labeled immunoglobulin antibotulinum toxin type A. Localization is around the spore coat and exosporium (f). An impermeable spore cortex (cx) is the limit of ferritin penetration. X52,000. From the work of J. J. Duda and J. M. Slack, *J. Bact.*, **97**:900, 1969.

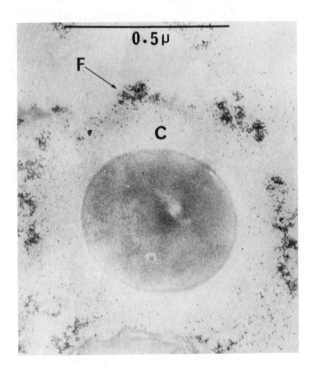

Fig. 3-14 Pneumococcus type A reacted with type specific ferritin-conjugated immunoglobulin *prior* to fixation, embedding, and sectioning. Ferritin (F) forms patchy precipitates on the swollen capsule (C). Not all the capsular surface is stained. The conjugate apparently fails to penetrate the interior of the swollen capsule. From the work of R. F. Baker and C. G. Loosli, *Lab. Invest.*, **15**: 716, 1966.

Fig. 3-15 Pneumococcus type I, glutaraldehyde fixed and embedded in low viscosity epon. Exposed *after* sectioning to type specific antiserum and the unlabeled antibody enzyme method (Chapter 6). The entire capsule is electron-opaque. There are no lucid spaces among opaque patches. There is no swelling of the capsule as the immunocytochemical reaction was carried out on the thin section of embedded organisms. X47,000. From the work of L. A. Sternberger.

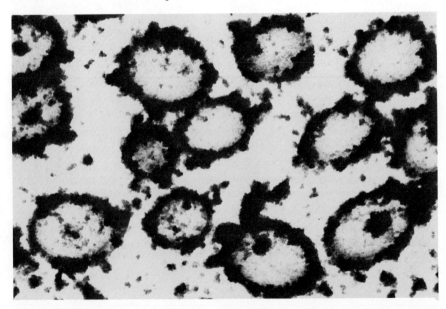

been thought to be associated with spore formation and not with the vegetative form. Indeed, ferritin-conjugated antitoxin type A did not localize onto type A *Clostridium botulinum* cells prior to the 20th hour of culture (Fig. 3-13).

The "Quellung" or swelling of the polysaccharide capsule of pneumococci with type specific antisera has long been known to be due to permeation of the reacting antibodies into the capsule and lattice formation with the polysaccharide. The increased volume of the capsule is thought to reflect the volume of the reacted antibody. Using ferritin-labeled immunoglobulin specific to type I polysaccharide, Baker and Loosli obtained with unfixed type-specific pneumococci only patchy localization on the surface of the capsule and none in its interior (Fig. 3-14). Localization of capsular polysaccharide is uniform upon immunostaining on the ultrathin section by another method (Fig. 3-15).

APPLICATION: THE INTERIOR OF CELLS IN SUSPENSION

Mammalian virology has been one of the chief benefactors of the immunoferritin technique. With viruses that cause acute disease, such as influenza, poliomyelitis, or smallpox, infection of host-homologous, established tissue culture cell lines usually leads to typical cytopathic effects. Early after ingestion of the virus by pinocytosis (e.g., vaccinia or reovirus), or membrane fusion (e.g., influenza, sendai, or vesicular stomatitis virus), cellular DNA and protein synthesis decline, while viral nucleotide kinases and nucleic acid polymerases and, eventually, virus constituents are synthesized with increasing rates. Concomitantly, there is vesiculation of the cytoplasm or nucleus, fragmentation of cell structure along with formation of new structures, some of which eventually assume the morphologic form of mature viral particles. When the process is slow, such as in the formation of vaccinia viruses, many morphologic stages can be distinguished. Disintegration of the infecting viruses, immature and mature particles of progeny viruses as well as their manner of secretion can be observed morphologically without immunocytochemical techniques. When the formation of progeny viruses is more rapid and the viruses are smaller, such changes are often more obscure. The progeny viruses seem to appear more precipitously as densely packed, crystalloid intracellular structures. This is typical of the intranuclear formation of adenoviruses. As the morphology of assembly is vague, immunocytochemistry has been increasingly important. Let us illustrate, therefore, the extensive contributions of the immunoferritin technique to virology by examples of such cytopathic viruses whose intracellular life cycle has been ill-defined by purely morphologic electron microscopy.

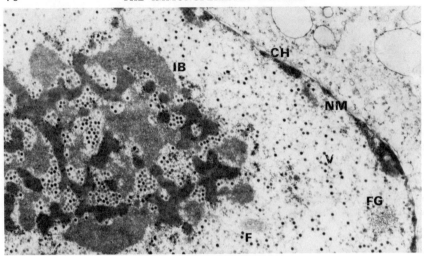

Fig. 3-16 Portion of an established human amniotic cell (line AV-3) infected with adenovirus type 12, not immunostained. Besides viral inclusion bodies (IB) and separate viral particles (V), bundles of fibers (F) and fibrogranular material (FG) have appeared in the infected nucleus. CH, marginal chromatin; NM, nuclear membrane. X10,000. From the work of H. F. Stich and co-workers, *J. Ultrastruct. Res.*, **19**:556, 1967.

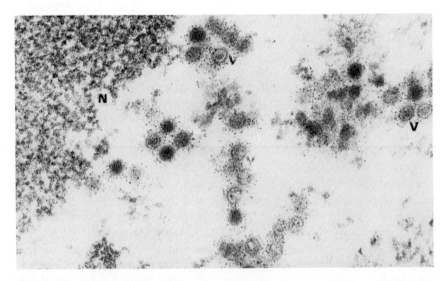

Fig. 3-17 Nucleus of human amniotic cells 48 hours after adenovirus 12 infection, treated with antiadenovirus serum and ferritin-conjugated antiglobulin. Ferritin is seen in association with the viral particles (V). The nuclear material itself (N) is free of ferritin. X55,000. From the work of H. F. Stich and co-workers, *J. Ultrastruct. Res.*, **19**:556, 1967.

The cytopathic effects may have been one of the greatest assists to the outstanding success of the immunoferritin applications to virology. Penetration of intracellular structures by labeled antibodies, which remains one of the major problems in the immunoferritin method, may have been minimized in a cell extensively damaged and vacuolated in the later stages of a cytopathic virus infection.

Cytopathy and viral replication is not a necessary result of viral infection. Instead, the virus may be incorporated into the genome of the cell. This incorporation may or may not be expressed by the surviving cell or its progeny. One form of expression is uncontrolled cell division, such as malignant transformation. The transformation may be associated with abnormal antigens as determined by immunocytochemistry. It is possible that the survival of these viruses is assured by the fact that under certain conditions (in certain tissues or hosts) they are cytopathic, while in other conditions they are oncogenic.

Adenovirus type 12 replicates rapidly in cytopathic infection of human amnion cells. A viral antigen (V antigen) is one of the virus-associated products of cell lysis and represents constituents of the protein coat of the virion. The virus causes tumors in hamsters. The tumors are free of V antigen. They do contain a tumor-associated antigen (T antigen) not found in normal hamster cells.

An amniotic cell contains in its nucleus late in the infectious cycle several new discernible structures besides a dense network of viral particles (Fig. 3-16). Upon use of the indirect method, viral antigen was found on the viral particles (Fig. 3-17) and viral inclusion bodies. The periphery of the inclusion bodies contained more ferritin than their central portions, apparently indicating incomplete penetration of the conjugate. Also, ferritin was seen in connection with ovoid electron-opaque areas surrounded by less opaque material (Fig. 3-18). The restriction of ferritin to the less opaque peripheral parts again suggests a problem of penetration. Finally, ferritin was seen in patches having no definite morphology. These were seen in the early stages of cell infection also and may represent nascent viruses. Only dense accumulations of ferritin particles are significant, since controls also had deposits, albeit weaker ones (Fig. 3-19).

Specifically deposited ferritin was conspicuously absent from nuclear structures, such as chromosomes, nucleoli, nuclear membrane, and nucleoplasm, and also from the bundles of fibers formed in the infected cell (Fig. 3-16). If staining with ferritin labeled anti-IgG is done after application of antiserum to T antigen, these fibers accept a heavy deposit of ferritin, while the structures stained after application of antiviral antiserum fail to stain.

Sometimes it is difficult to decide whether lack of staining of a structure by ferritin-conjugated antibody is due to lack of antigen or lack of

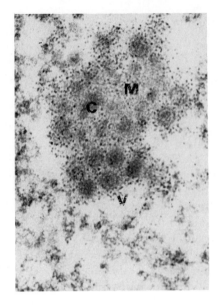
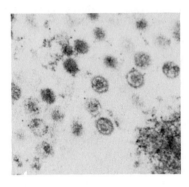

Fig. 3-18   Fig. 3-19

Fig. 3-18   Another portion of a nucleus of a cell similar to that in Fig. 3-18 containing ovoid, electron-opaque clumps (C) that are surrounded with a less opaque matrix (M). Ferritin particles are in association with the matrix and nearby viral particles (V). X68,500. From the work of H. F. Stich and co-workers, *J. Ultrastruct. Res., 19:556, 1967.*

Fig. 3-19   Portion of a nucleus of an infected cell similar to those in Figs. 3-16 to 3-18 exposed to normal rabbit immunoglobulin and ferritin-labeled antiimmunoglobulin. The occasional deposit of ferritin granules in controls (page 84) are characteristic in staining of intracellular antigens by the immunoferritin technique. Such nonspecific staining raises the "noise" level and limits the method to abundant antigens and to high titered antisera, at least when intracellular antigens are investigated. X56,200. From the work of H. F. Stich and co-workers, *J. Ultrastruct. Res., 19:556, 1967.*

penetration. If the unstained structure is closely associated with a stained one, sonication of the cell may resolve the problem. For instance, tobacco etch virus infection stimulates formation of cylindrical inclusion bodies in infected leaves. Staining of sonicates with ferritin-labeled purified antiviral antibodies showed that the inclusions are distinct from the virus itself and that, contrary to previous thinking, the inclusions do not represent viral coat protein (Fig. 3-20).

The replication of RNA (reo) and DNA (vaccinia) viruses in the cytoplasm of L-cells has been studied by Dales and co-workers, using nucleotide-labeled inoculum viruses. Uptake of virus is by phagocytosis. In the case of reoviruses, 15% of the RNA label is found in the foci of progeny virus morphogenesis. These foci of virus inclusions occur in close association with the spindle tubules of the host cell (Fig. 3-8). The

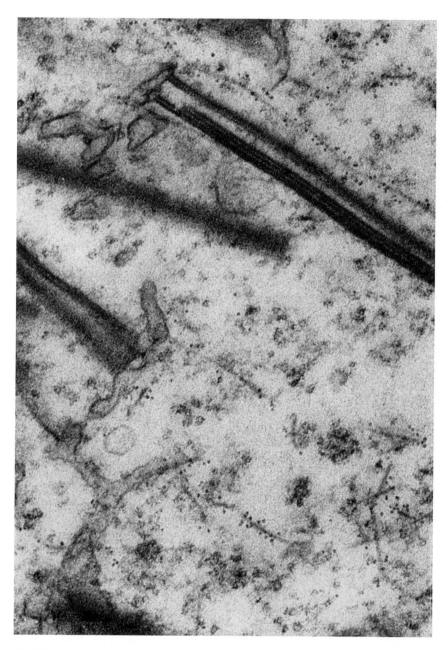

Fig. 3-20 Tobacco etch virus infection. The viral aggregates are localized by ferritin-conjugated antibody. The adjacent, electron-opaque, cylindrical inclusions are associated with the endoplasmic reticulum and are free of ferritin. X135,000. From the work of J. F. Shepard and T. A. Shalla, *Virology,* **38**:186, 1969.

periphery of the viral particles is tagged with ferritin. Particles in the interior as well as the exterior of the inclusion accept the ferritin label. The penetration of the label to this location has probably been facilitated by the digitonin pretreatment of the cell (page 70). The mitotic spindle is also specifically stained with ferritin-antibody conjugate. The spindle tubules fail to form when the cell is treated with colchicine, a procedure that leaves viral replication unaffected. Hence, despite their specific tagging these structures are not necessary for viral replication. On the other hand, kinky filaments that are seen in lucid zones in the aggregates of viral particles in the inclusion are always seen in conjunction with viral replication and appear to be essential. The filaments are devoid, however, of viral antigen as evident by lack of ferritin tagging.

APPLICATION: THE INTERIOR OF SOLID TISSUES

Successful control of the problem of penetration into the interior of the cell is illustrated by studies of H. Tanaka and D. H. Moore on the localization of antigens of mammary tumors. There are two morphologically slightly dissimilar viral particles associated with the acinar tumor cell (an acinus is a lumen surrounded by an epithelial wall). *A* particles are in the cytoplasm of the cell, and *B* particles are in the lumen. The ferritin-conjugated rabbit IgG anti-mammary mouse tumor (from milk of strain R III) has been freed of unconjugated IgG by *repeated* ultracentrifugations and has been absorbed with rat liver powder, and with C57 BC mouse tissue and milk powder (C57 BC mice are free of mammary tumor virus). To assure penetration of conjugate, tissue has to be subjected to fixation in cold 5% formalin and extensive rinsing, grinding, freezing, and thawing. Ferritin-antibody is localized only on the budding *B* particles and those found in the acinar lumen (Fig. 3-21). This restricted localization to the surface of the cell is not due to lack of penetrability of the cell, because unabsorbed conjugate gives extensive nonspecific localization, and this localization occurs throughout the cytoplasm.

INTERPRETATION OF IMMUNOFERRITIN STAINING

On sections counterstained with lead, ferritin granules are not the only opaque granules. Chromatin components and ribosomes, for instance, are equally opaque. Fortunately, the submolecular structure of ferritin permits differentiation from these opacities. Ferritin-conjugated antibodies could, therefore, be used to identify and quantitate antigenic determinants on single molecules if the method were free of factors that reduce the *specificity* of staining, that prevent equal *accessibility* of all subcellular

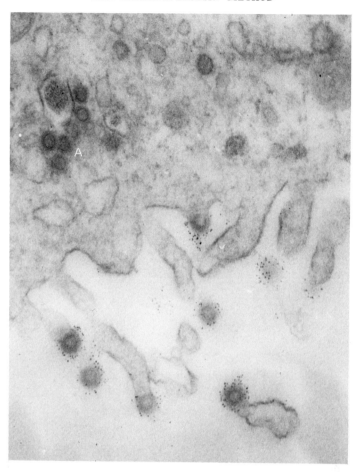

Fig. 3-21 Mouse mammary tumor (RIII strain) stained with ferritin-conjugated IgG antimouse mammary tumor. The intracellular viral A particles (A) are unstained. Only the mature B particles when budding at the cell membrane into the acinar lumen assume the antigen, which tags with ferritin-conjugated antibodies. The budding B particles have acquired viral antigens different from those of the host cell even in the very early stages of the budding process. This sequence of acquisition of ferritin-antibody-reactive antigen during budding is similar to that of myxoviruses. From H. Tanaka and D. H. Moore, *Virology*, **33:**197, 1967.

tissue components to the conjugate, and that prevent *interference of localization* by unconjugated antibody.

Specificity of staining

In ferritin-conjugated antibody the ferritin molecule bears many carbamido-bonded substituents of which usually only one has reacted with antibody. The others are carbamidotoluene amine groups [several of the groups shown in Fig. 3-4(d) attached to a ferritin molecule]. We have seen that in the case of fluorescent antibodies a reliable and specific conjugate has been prepared only when it had been realized that not more than one to two fluorescent groups should be conjugated per molecule of antibody. In the ferritin method the severity of excessive substitution in the ferritin molecule can be alleviated by using a mild conjugation reaction, such as that described above (page 67) and by absorbing the conjugate with tissue powder prior to staining (such as in the work of Tanaka and Moore, page 82). However, in most of the published use of ferritin-antibody conjugates, these two precautions have not been taken. Neither should one expect that absorption with tissue powder will make the immunoferritin conjugate entirely specific, since similar procedures have been unreliable in immunofluorescence in the prechromatography days.

Poor specificity of immunoferritin staining expresses itself most often in the interior of the cell upon staining prior to embedding. When specific staining under these conditions is extensive, controls may reveal a lesser number, but not absence of ferritin particles. Only when specific localization is sparse can absence of ferritin in controls be expected.

Although conjugation itself favors aggregation of single ferritin with single immunoglobulin molecules by covalent bonding, staining of the cell surface by the direct method often suggests noncovalent formation of larger aggregates. Just as the nonspecific staining, this aggregation may be due to the polarity of the conjugated ferritin surface. The localization of ferritin is patchy on the surface of the capsule of the pneumococcus in Fig. 3-14, even though the actual distribution of polysaccharide antigen extends over the entire periphery of the capsule as a continuum (Fig. 3-15). The patchiness of ferritin is, therefore, not due to a patchy distribution of the antigen but rather to clumping of the conjugate itself.

Ferritin-conjugated immunoglobulin anti-sheep erythrocyte (anti-SRBC), at a concentration four times higher than its agglutination titer, gives patchy localization on the cell surface and forms bridges between the aggregated cells (Fig. 3-1), ranging from 50–90 nm in width. The distance between the two N-terminal ends on the FAb fragment of IgG is about 14 nm in the normal state. The distance could conceivably be increased to about 17 nm, if the molecule were stretched as it may be when each of the FAb portions attaches to adjacent cells and agglutinates them by an antibody bridge. The conjugation of a ferritin molecule to IgG does not increase the maximum distance between the FAb portions. Hence, the bridges in Fig. 3-1 cannot be formed by conjugates of a single ferritin with a single antibody molecule, but must have been the result of aggregation of the ferritin conjugate. Comparison with Figs. 4-8, 4-9, and 4-10 shows that with the use of other methods the expected dimensions of antibody-bridged cell surfaces prevail.

A suggestion of noncovalent aggregation of ferritin-immunoglobulin conjugates is also apparent from the work of Fresen and Vogt in which hemolytic activity of immunoglobulin anti-SRBC was reduced 16-fold by conjugation. Extensive washing of the cells after reaction with conjugate restored the hemolytic titer to ¼ of that of unconjugated immunoglobulin. Apparently, nonspecific material that contributed towards steric hindrance was removed during washing.

At high resolution the morphology of labeling may itself suggest a way of differentiating between specific and nonspecific localization, as proposed by Dales. When the structure that is specifically tagged by ferritin-antibody is well defined, such as a viral particle or a cell membrane, the clusters of ferritin are separated by a lucid zone from the localized structure. In specific staining this lucid zone is not wider than 8 nm. The width is the sum of the distance of the core from the surface of the ferritin molecule and of the point of conjugation of the ferritin molecule with antibody from the specific antibody combining site. When a structure is nonspecifically stained this distance is invariably less, so much so that the ferritin appears to be localized directly on the membrane. Apparently, in nonspecific localization it is the free ferritin or the ferritin moiety of the conjugate that attaches to a structure and not the antibody moiety of the conjugate. This again suggests that nonspecific localization is a property of ferritin and not of immunoglobulin and may be due to polar substituents on the ferritin molecules.

Accessibility of antigen to ferritin-immunoglobulin conjugates

Even supposedly homogeneous matrices, penetrable to unlabeled antibodies are apparently inaccessible to ferritin-immunoglobulin conjugate. Thus, only the periphery of the swelled pneumococcal capsule is stained with specific ferritin-antibody conjugate (Fig. 3-14). On the other hand, the antibody reagents of the unlabeled antibody enzyme method (Chapter 6) stain the whole thickness of the swelled capsule on application to suspended cells, indicating that antibodies penetrate well. Thus, failure of penetration of the ferritin-immunoglobulin conjugate is probably not only due to the increase in size of the immunoglobulin molecule (maximal diameter 14 nm), resulting from conjugation with one ferritin molecule (diameter 12 nm). The diameter of the largest molecules in such a conjugate would not exceed 26 nm, while many molecular species may be smaller depending on the site of attachment of ferritin to immunoglobulin. Such conjugate molecules are not significantly larger than peroxidase-antiperoxidase complex (diameter

21 nm) that penetrates the capsule with ease. The difficulty of penetration of the ferritin-immunoglobulin conjugate is probably again the result of nonspecific aggregation.

When sheep red cells are stained by the indirect ferritin-antibody method (unlabeled rabbit serum anti-SRBC followed by ferritin-conjugated immunoglobulin anti-rabbit IgG) agglutination of the cells by the unlabeled antiserum largely prevents, in the work of H Schäfer, the accessibility of the labeled antibody. On the other hand, peroxidase-antiperoxidase complex penetrates easily into the interspaces of agglutinated SRBC, staining the cell surface as a continuum (Fig. 7-1). Apparently in the case of ferritin antibodies, again we are dealing with secondary aggregates of a conjugate.

Interference of localization

Incomplete removal of unlabeled antibody may interfere with the localization of intracellular antigens by ferritin-antibody conjugates. Unlabeled antibody penetrates the cell faster than labeled material. Its earlier arrival at a subcellular site may block staining of the slower diffusing conjugate. Thus, a small amount of unlabeled antibody may effectively hinder the staining with a larger amount of conjugated antibody. The pneumococcal capsule (Fig. 3-14) again illustrates this situation. The capsule is swelled because of the effect of specific antibodies that interspace themselves into the capsular matrix as antigen-antibody precipitates. Apparently, the unlabeled antibodies that contaminate the ferritin-immunoglobulin conjugate penetrate the capsule rapidly, causing its swelling prior to the arrival of the conjugate. Any conjugate that does penetrate diffuses at a slower rate and finds sites in the interior of the capsule blocked by unlabeled antibody. At the surface of the capsule, however, conjugated and unconjugated antibodies are able to compete effectively for antigen since both react simultaneously. Hence, staining by ferritin remains limited to the capsular surface. The presence of unlabeled antibodies may also be responsible for the patchy localization of anti-SRBC antibodies on the surface of sheep red cells (Fig. 3-1), a location known by other methods to possess continuous antigen (Fig. 7-1).

In the indirect method unlabeled antibodies are probably no significant impediment to efficient staining of surface-localized antigen. Since an antibody molecule localized in the first step of the indirect method reacts in the second step with several anti-IgG molecules, chances are high that in most cases at least one conjugate molecule or aggregate reacts with a localized antibody molecule.

The overall evidence suggests that the difficulties in specificity and penetration of ferritin-immunoglobulin conjugates are due to the process of conjugation itself. They are not primarily a property of the native ferritin molecule. Avoidance of conjugation altogether and specific attachment of native, unaltered ferritin to the antigen site by noncovalent bonds appears to be a logical solution of this problem and is discussed in the next chapter.

REFERENCES

Andres, G. A., Accinni, L., Hsu, K. C., Zabricskie, J. B., and Seegal, B. J. Electron microscopic studies of human glomerulonephritis with ferritin-conjugated antibody. Localization of antigen antibody complexes in glomerular structures of patients with acute glomerulonephritis. *J. Exp. Med.*, 123:399, 1966.

Baker, R. F. and Loosli, C. G. The ultrastructure of encapsulated *Diplococcus pneumoniae* type I before and after exposure to type specific antibody. *Lab. Invest.*, 15:716, 1966.

Birnbaum, U., Vogt, A., and Marinis, S. Isolation and characterization of immunoferritin conjugates. II. Antibody binding capacity *in vitro*. *Immunology*, 18:443, 1970.

Dales, S., Gomatos, P. J., and Hsu, K. C. The uptake and development of reovirus in strain L-cells followed with labeled viral ribonucleic acid and ferritin-antibody conjugates. *Virology*, 25:193, 1965.

Davis, W. Z., Douglas, S. S., Petz, L. D., and Fudenberg, H. H. Ferritin-antibody localization of erythrocyte antigenic sites in immune hemolytic anemia. *J. Immunol.*, 101:621, 1968.

Douglas, S. D., Gottlieb, A. J., Strauss, A. J. L., and Spicer, S. S. Selectivity of ferritin-protein conjugates for sites on skeletal muscle. *Exp. Mol. Path.*, Suppl. 3:5, 1966.

Duda, J. J. and Slack, J. M. Toxin production in *Clostridium botulinum* as demonstrated by electron microscopy. *J. Bacteriology*, 97:900, 1969.

Fresen, K. O. and Vogt, A. The hemolytic activity of ferritin-labeled antibodies against sheep erythrocytes. *Med. Biol. Immunol.*, 157:24, 1971.

Gracea, E., Voiculescu, R., Zarnea, G., Ionescu, M., and Botez, D. Electron microscopic study of phase I and II. *C. burneti* in the chick yolk sack by use of ferritin conjugated antibody. *Z. Immunitätsf.*, 140:358, 1970.

Howe, C., Spiler, H., Minio, F., and Hsu, K. Z. Electron microscopic study of erythrocyte receptors with labeled antisera to membrane components. *J. Immunol.*, 104:1406, 1970.

Mardiney, M. R., Müller-Eberhard, N. J., and Feldman, J. D. Ultrastructural localization of the third and fourth component of complement on complement cell complexes. *Am. J. Path.*, **53**:253, 1968.

Marinis, S., Vogt, A., and Brandner, G. Isolation and characterization of immunoferritin conjugates. I. The molecular ratio. *Immunology*, **17**:77, 1969.

Pierce, T. B., Ram, J. S., and Midgley, A. R. Labeled antibodies in electron microscopy. *Int. Rev. Exp. Path.*, **3**:1, 1964.

Schäfer, H. *Immunoelectron microscopy*, Gustav Fischer Verlag, Stuttgart, 1971.

Shepard, J. F. and Shella, T. A. Tobacco etch virus cylindrical inclusions: Antigenically unrelated to the causal virus. *Virology*, **38**:186, 1969.

Singer, S. J. and Schick, A. F. The properties of specific stains for electron microscopy prepared by conjugation of antibody molecules with ferritin. *J. Biophys. Biochem. Cytol.*, **9**:519, 1961.

Sternberger, L. A. Electron microscopic immunocytochemistry: A review. *J. Histochem. Cytochem.*, **15**:139, 1967.

Stich, H. F., Kalnins, V. I., MacKinnon, E., and Yohn, B. S. Electron microscopic localization of adenovirus type 12 antigen. *J. Ultrastruct. Res.*, **19**:556, 1967.

Tanaka, H. The ferritin-labeled antibody method: its advantages and disadvantages. A methodological review. *Acta Haematol. Japonica*, **31**:125, 1968.

Tanaka, H. and Moore, D. H. Electron microscopic localization of viral antigen in mouse mammary tumors by ferritin-labeled antibodies. *Virology*, **33**:197, 1967.

Vogt, A., Bockhorn, H., Kozina, K., and Sasaki, M. Electron microscopic localization of nephrotoxic antibodies in the glomeruli of the rat after intravenous application of purified nephritogenic antibody-ferritin conjugates. *J. Exp. Med.*, **127**:867, 1968.

Vogt, A. and Kopp, R. Loss of specific agglutinating activity of purified ferritin-conjugated antibodies. *Nature*, **202**:1350, 1964.

Wagner, M. and Veckenstedt, A. Electron microscopic detection of mengovirus in L-cells with ferritin-labeled antibody. *Arch. Gesamte Virusforsch.*, **32**:147, 1970.

Chapter 4

The Hybrid Antibody Method

In any single antibody molecule each of the light chains and each of the heavy chains is identical. It follows that both specific combining sites in an IgG molecule are identical. Despite extensive search, no antibodies have been found in nature that by virtue of a dual specificity could cross-link different antigens. Such antibodies can, however, be prepared in the laboratory. Their use has been introduced into immunocytochemistry by U. Hämmerling, T. Aoki, Etienne de Harven, E. A. Boyse, and L. J. Old. An antibody with dual specificity with one combining site specific for a tissue antigen, such as vesicular stomatitis virus (VSV), and the other site specific for an electron histochemical detector, such as ferritin, would make a clean reagent for attaching ferritin onto VSV and detecting the viral antigen without use of covalently labeled antibody reagents.

We have seen earlier (page 7) that digestion of IgG with pepsin degrades the bulk of the Fc region into dialyzable fragments but leaves the hinge region and the Fab regions intact. At least one of the interchain disulfide bonds at the hinge region is maintained and, therefore, the Fab fragments do not fall apart. The antibody fragment [$F(ab')_2$] is still divalent and precipitates with multivalent antigens. The inter-H-chain disulfide bond is, however, unusually exposed and more susceptible to reduction than the intrachain disulfide bonds and the single L-H chain interchain disulfide bond in each Fab portion of the antibody fragment. Consequently, mild reduction cleaves the bivalent fragment, $F(ab')_2$ into two identical monovalent fragments, Fab′. These fragments combine with specific antigen and inhibit precipitation of the antigen with undigested, homologous antibody. Upon removal of the reducing agent, the Fab′ fragments reoxidize, and the $F(ab')_2$ is reconstituted (Fig. 4-1).

The homology of reconstitution is low: specific Fab′ in a mixture of heterologous Fab′ favors recombination with its own specific kind only slightly over recombination with any other Fab′. Thus, if a mixture of Fab′ anti-VSV and Fab′ antiferritin is allowed to reoxidize, some of the recombinants will be $F(ab')_2$, possessing one combining site reactive with VSV

89

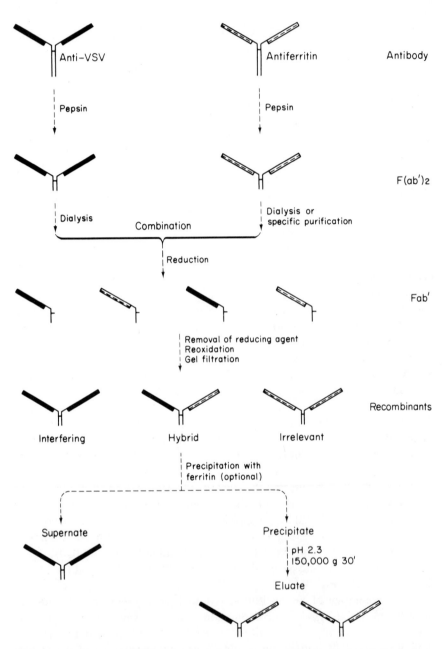

Fig. 4-1 Preparation of hybrid antivesicular stomatitis virus (VSV)/antiferritin antibody from IgG anti-VSV and IgG antiferritin.

and another with ferritin [F(ab')$_2$ anti-VSV/antiferritin]. When application of these recombinants to VSV antigen in tissue is followed by ferritin, regularly spaced specific deposition of ferritin is observed.

Besides hybrid recombinants, homospecific recombinants form. If a mixture of digested purified anti-VSV and antiferritin is reduced and reoxidized, these homospecific recombinants will be bivalent anti-VSV and bivalent antiferritin. The antiferritin is inconsequential as it is washed away during cytochemical staining. The anti-VSV, however, will interfere with the localization of the hybrid antibody and, thus, with the localization of ferritin.

The interfering recombinants (anti-VSV/anti-VSV in our example) can be separated by immunospecific purification from the hybrid antibody (anti-VSV/antiferritin) and the antiferritin homospecific recombinants (antiferritin/antiferritin).

Specific purification may be omitted if the proportion of anti-VSV/anti-VSV in the recombinant mixture is minimized. This can be done by increasing the proportion of F(ab')$_2$ antiferritin to F(ab')$_2$ anti-VSV during reduction and oxidation.

If equal amount of purified F(ab')$_2$ antiferritin and anti-VSV are admixed during reduction and if oxidative recombination is random, one would expect to obtain 50% anti-VSV/antiferritin, 25% antiferritin/antiferritin, and 25% anti-VSV/anti-VSV. On the other hand, if four parts of purified F(ab')$_2$ antiferritin are admixed with one part of purified F(ab')$_2$ anti-VSV, one would expect 32% anti-VSV/antiferritin, 64% antiferritin/antiferritin, and 4% anti-VSV/anti-VSV. Thus, the proportion of the interfering anti-VSV/anti-VSV is greatly reduced, while the theoretical yield of hybrid anti-VSV/antiferritin is reduced only moderately.

If four parts of purified F(ab')$_2$ antiferritin are hybridized with one part of non-purified F(ab')$_2$ from IgG anti-VSV and if $\frac{1}{6}$ of the IgG is anti-VSV, then one would expect 5% anti-VSV/antiferritin, 94% irrelevant recombinants, and 1% interfering anti-VSV/anti-VSV and anti-VSV/nonspecific Fab'. Thus, failure to purify anti-VSV although reducing the yield of useful hybrid antibody has the salutary effect of also reducing interfering recombinants, although not to the same extent. If neither the anti-VSV nor the antiferritin is purified and if we assume that $\frac{1}{6}$ of the IgG antiferritin is specific antiferritin, then we would expect 1% anti-VSV/anti-ferritin, 91% irrelevant recombinants, and 8% interfering anti-VSV/anti-VSV and anti-VSV/nonspecific Fab'. Failure to use purified antiferritin has further reduced the yield of anti-VSV/antiferritin hybrid and has increased the proportion of interfering recombinants. The reason for the increase of interfering recombinants is that now the IgG antiferritin supplies a large proportion of nonspecific Fab' that forms interfering recombinants with the Fab' anti-VSV. Nevertheless, as we shall see, the use of purified antiferritin may not necessarily be advisable.

The above calculations are based on random recombination of Fab' fragments. In fact there exists some homology in the recombining hinge region that results in some degree of homing of the fragments, thus, increasing the proportion of homoligated recombinants and decreasing the yield of desired hybrid approximately by another 50%.

PREPARATION OF HYBRID ANTIBODIES: PROCEDURE

We will illustrate the procedure by the preparation of directly reacting antivesicular stomatitis virus (VSV)/antiferritin hybrid antibody for the localization of the VSV outer coat antigen on cell surfaces. Solutions in acetate buffer, pH 4.5, of 10 mg per ml of IgG anti-VSV and 10 mg per ml of IgG antiferritin are digested *separately* with 0.2 mg/ml of pepsin for 20 hours at 37°. Reaction is terminated by adjustment to pH 8.0 with sodium hydroxide. Small peptides are removed by dialysis against 0.5 M acetate buffer, pH 5.0, at 4°. Two mg anti-VSV digest, and 8 mg antiferritin digest [F(ab')$_2$] are mixed, and 2-mercaptoethylamine is added under nitrogen to a concentration of 0.015 M. After one hour at 37° the solution is passed through a 10 × 120 mm cation exchange column at pH 5.0 (AG 50W-X4). The eluted protein is adjusted to pH 8.0 with sodium hydroxide and reoxidized while stirring in an oxygen atmosphere for six hours. Following concentration by vacuum filtration, the solution is passed through a Sephadex-G100 column equilibriated with Tris buffer, pH 8.6, containing 0.2 M sodium chloride. The frontally eluted protein peak fractions are concentrated, sterilized by passage through a membrane filter, and stored at 4°.

Instead of IgG, purified anti-VSV and antiferritin could be employed, or the purification can be done after pepsin digestion and neutralization to pH 8.0. The latter is preferred, because it can replace the dialysis step. Additional specific purification with ferritin after oxidative recombination removes hybrid antibodies along with antiferritin/antiferritin and antiferritin/nonspecific Fab' recombinants from other recombinants. If this additional purification is contemplated, it is more efficient to admix 8 mg rather than 2mg of the anti-VSV digest with 8 mg antiferritin digest.

For the purification of IgG or F(ab')$_2$ antiferritin or of hybrid antibody relatively rich in antiferritin/antiferritin recombinants, add a slight excess of ferritin, incubate at room temperature for one hour, and leave at 1° for two days. Centrifuge at 1,000 g and wash precipitate in saline three times. Resuspend precipitate and adjust to pH 2.3 at 1°. Irrespective of whether or not the precipitate dissolves completely, recentrifuge the suspension or solution, as the case may be, at 150,000 g at 1° for 30 minutes, and collect, and neutralize the colorless supernatant layer of purified antiferritin.

If the hybrid antibody preparation is relatively poor in antiferritin/anti-ferritin recombinants, addition of slight excess of ferritin may result in only incomplete coprecipitation of hybrid antiferritin. In this case leave the mixture of hybrid antibody preparation and ferritin at 1–5° for one hour and centrifuge at 150,000 g at 1° for 30 minutes. Remove the supernatant colorless layer and wash the sediment and the brown liquid on the bottom of the tube in saline three times. Resuspend and proceed with the acid treatment as above.

The hybrid antibody method, of course, is not limited to ferritin as a marker. The F(ab')$_2$ antiferritin could be replaced with F(ab')$_2$ specific to a cytochemically detectable enzyme (page 110) and the hybrid antibody be used to link the enzyme to a specific antigen site. Purification of the recombinants, if desired, could be done by immunoabsorbents. The alternative purification based on specific precipitation with soluble enzyme, dissociation at acid pH, and separation of enzyme and recombinants by sedimentation would not be as simple as in the case of ferritin-recombinant complexes, since the smaller molecular weight difference of the enzyme and the recombinants requires separation by zonal gradients. Also in the case of peroxidase, one has to contend with a low dissociability of avid antibody from antigen, even at acid pH (page 131). Therefore when purification of the product is contemplated, high molecular weight markers are preferred in the hybrid antibody method. In addition to ferritin, such markers are provided by some of the smaller viruses as for example southern bean mosaic virus (SMBV) introduced by Ulrich Hämmerling and his associates (Figs. 4–2 and 4–3). Viruses are often so compact that they can be readily recognized in the electron microscope despite an elemental composition similar to that of mammalian tissue. Recognition is especially easy on the cell surface because of lack of surrounding opaque structures such as ribosomes. The hybrid antibody method has been exclusively used for detection

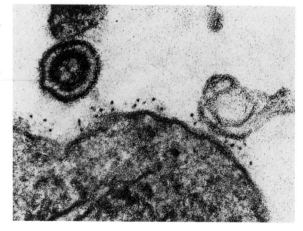

Fig. 4-2 Identification of Gross antigen on C57BL leukemia cells induced by Gross virus. Mouse anti-Gross leukemia serum followed by anti-IgG/antiferritin hybrid antibody and ferritin. The cells were fixed after immunostaining in 1% glutaraldehyde and 1% buffered osmium tetroxide, counterstained with uranyl acetate and embedded with Epon. Patches of the cell surface are labeled. The Gross virus is unlabeled. X156,000. From T. Aoki, F. M. Booyse, L. J. Old, E. de Harven, U. Hämmerling, and H. A. Wood, *Proc. Nat. Acad. Sci., U.S.,* **56**:569, 1970.

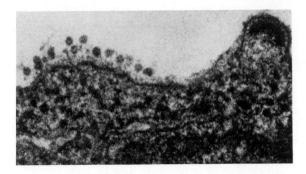

Fig. 4-3 Similar results are obtained by staining with anti-Gross leukemia serum followed by anti-IgG/antisouthern bean mosaic virus (SMBV) hybrid antibody and SMBV. X156,000. From T. Aoki, E. A. Booyse, L. J. Old, E. de Harven, U. Hämmerling, and H. A. Wood, Proc. Nat. Acad. Sci., U.S., 65:569, 1970.

of antigen on the cell surface. The morphologic dissimilarity of SBMV and ferritin permits differentiation of two antigens on the cell surface in the same preparation.

DIRECT STAINING WITH NONPURIFIED HYBRID ANTIBODIES

In our discussion of ferritin-labeled antibodies, we encountered viruses, such as vaccinia or reovirus, that enter the host cell via phagocytosis. In this process the viral core is liberated by lysosomal uncoating in the phagocytic vacuole. On purely morphologic evidence it has been suspected that membrane-enclosed viruses, such as influenza, Sendai, and vesicular stomatitis virus (VSV), enter the cell by fusion of their membranes with that of the host cell followed by release of the viral nucleoprotein directly into the host cell cytoplasm. However, a high multiplicity of infecting viral particles relative to the number of cells studied is needed in order to insure that a thin section of the cell contains a viral particle with reasonable probability. Since the host cell in culture is continually in the process of phagocytosis (pinocytosis), some particles of necessity will be found in phagocytic vacuoles after high multiplicity infection whether or not this is the normal infective pathway. To ascertain membrane fusion as the sole mechanism of infection, it is necessary to show that the viral membrane actually becomes incorporated into the cell membrane and that, furthermore, none of the viral membrane proteins enter the cytoplasm. Evidence of the former can be obtained by preembedding staining electron immunocytochemistry. This has been provided by J. Heine and C. Schnaitman for vesicular stomatitis (VSV) using hybrid antibodies. Evidence of the latter cannot be provided by preembedding staining electron microscopy, because negative results may indicate failure of penetration of antibody reagents into the cell rather than absence of antigen in the cytoplasm. Therefore, the viral particle was labeled with ^{3}H-thymidine and ^{3}H-lysine. After infection of the cell at 4° and incubation at 37° for 15 minutes, a large proportion of viral nucleoprotein, but only an insignificant amount of viral membrane protein (separated by acrylamide gel electrophoresis), was found in the soluble cytoplasmic fraction, thus providing evidence that the viral core had degraded, while the membrane protein never entered the cell.

For electron immunocytochemistry of the viral membrane proteins, anti-VSV/antiferritin hybrid antibody was prepared by digestion of IgG fractions. The recombinants were *not* immunospecifically purified. Suspension-grown L-cells were infected in the cold and, after various periods of incubation at 37°, were washed in the cold and treated in an ice bath for 20 minutes with 0.25 mg of hybrid antibody preparation per 10^6 cells in a volume of 0.1 ml phosphate buffered saline (PBS) containing sucrose. Following two washings in PBS, the cells were treated for 30 minutes at 0° with 0.125 mg ferritin dissolved in PBS, washed twice, fixed in glutaraldehyde, and embedded for electron microscopy.

Free virus particles attached to the cell membrane can be seen if the cell is processed in the cold after infection in the cold without intervening incubation at 37° (Figs. 4-4 and 4-5). The hybrid antibody deposits an uninterrupted envelope of ferritin onto the surface of the viral particles. The ferritin coat is of rather uniform thickness.

After 10 minutes of incubation at 37°, viral particles are no longer morphologically discernible. Viral antigen, however, is now incorporated in the cell membrane proper (Fig. 4-6).

The distribution of antigen-bearing patches is spotty with some pref-

---

Figs. 4-4 and 4-5 **Fig. 4-4** Longitudinal section of vesicular stromatitis virus (VSV) stained with anti-VSV/antiferritin hybrid antibody and ferritin. X230,000. From J. W. Heine and C. A. Schnaitman, *J. Virol.*, 8:786, 1971. **Fig. 4-5** Transverse section stained as in Fig. 4-4. X230,000. From J. W. Heine and C. A. Schnaitman, *J. Virol.*, 8:786, 1971.

Fig. 4-4   **Fig. 4-5**

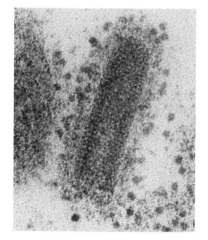

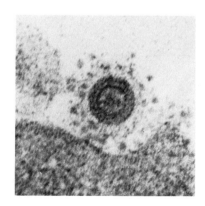

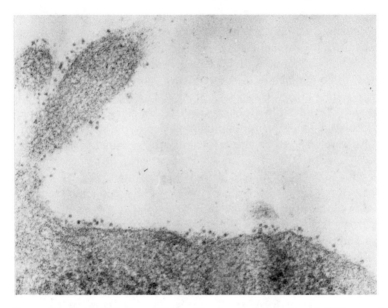

Fig. 4-6 L-cells, incubated at 37° for 10 min after adsorption of VSV, treated with anti-VSV/antiferritin hybrid antibody and ferritin. The cell membrane is stained in patches. X119,500. From J. W. Heine and C. A. Schnaitman, *J. Virol.,* **8:**786, 1971.

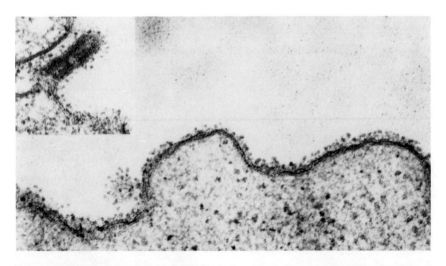

Fig. 4-7 Eight hours after infection VSV buds from the cell surface. Both the virion (inset) and the entire cell membrane accept the hybrid antibody in a continuous fashion. X105,000. From R. R. Wagner, J. W. Heine, G. Goldstein, and C. A. Schnaitman, *J. Virol.,* **7:**274, 1971.

erence for cellular processes. There is considerable variability in the amount of label on the cell surface proper. The labeling of the cell surface in spots shows that, indeed, the viral envelope is incorporated into the cell membrane. The total evidence indicates that vesicular stomatitis virus is incorporated into the cell by membrane fusion and not by phagocytosis.

Cells harvested eight hours after infection reveal budding progeny virus on their surfaces (Fig. 4-7). Hybrid antibody deposits ferritin granules over the entire viral as well as cellular surface.

The continuous distribution of label on the viral particle and on the cell membrane during viral release indicates that the patchy distribution seen on the cell membrane during initial stages of infection is real and not an artifact produced by the hybrid antibody as used.

Direct Staining with Hybrid Antibodies Prepared from Purified Antiferritin

Ferritin-*labeled* IgG antirabbit small intestinal sucrase-isomaltase localizes the entire luminal surface of enterocytes (Fig. 4-8). Labeling is more pronounced after tryptic digestion of the enteric surface coat. This and the

Fig. 4-8 Longitudinal section of a trypsin-treated enterocyte brush border region stained with ferritin-conjugated antisucrase. Ferritin is seen over most of the surface of the microvillar membrane. X44,000. From R. Gitzelmann, T. H. Bächli, H. Binz, J. Lindenmann, and G. Semenza, *Biochim. Biophys. Acta,* 196:20, 1970

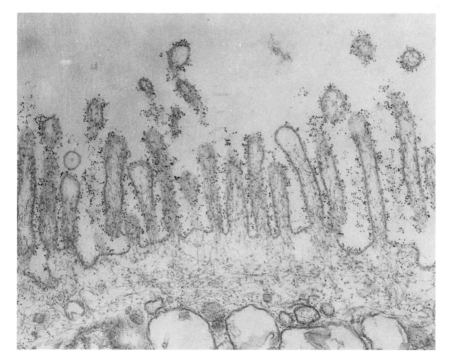

close approximation of ferritin to the surface suggests that sucrose forms an integral part of the outermost layer of the cell membrane. There is, however, considerable variation of the distance of individual ferritin particles from the site of attachment of labeled antibodies (see Fig. 3-1 and page 84). Use of hybrid antibodies offers opportunity to attain a more regular distance between ferritin granules and antigen sites. A regular distance is expected, because in the direct hybrid antibody method one ferritin molecule corresponds to a single antigen site, while in the ferritin-labeled antibody method the number of ferritin molecules per antigen site is variable. In the hybrid antibody method ferritin always attaches at the Fab′ antibody combining site, while in the ferritin-labeled method ferritin may be attached anywhere on the IgG surface. The only factor that can change the distance of ferritin to antigen in the hybrid antibody method is flexibility in the hinge region of $F(ab')_2$.

Knüsel, Bächli, Gitzelmann, and Lindenmann find, indeed, that in the intervillar spaces the ferritin molecules are regularly distributed by the hybrid antibody method (Fig. 4-9) but not by the ferritin-labeled antibody method (Fig. 4-8). In fact with the hybrid antibody method, the core of the ferritin molecules is equidistant from two apposing microvillar surfaces. If the diameter of ferritin is taken as 12 nm, the space between the cell surface and the ferritin surface is 5 nm, which is the expected space to accommodate a bent $F(ab')_2$ antibody fragment (Fig. 4-10).

In this work the antisucrase/antiferritin hybrid antibody has been prepared by the procedure essentially as outlined above for anti-VSV/anti-

Fig. 4-9 Longitudinal section of a trypsin-treated enterocyte brush border region stained with antisucrase/antiferritin hybrid antibody and ferritin. X75,000. Ferritin is deposited only on apposing surfaces. From A. Knüsel, T. H. Bächli, R. Gitzelmann, and J. Lindenmann, J. Immunol., 106:583, 1971.

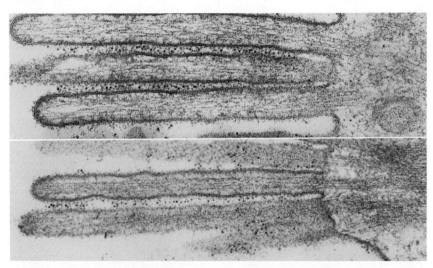

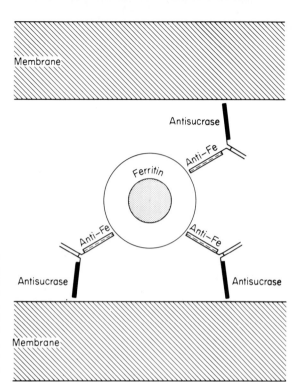

Fig. 4-10 Schematic representation of intervillar localization of ferritin by binding with several antiintestinal sucrase/antiferritin hybrid antibody molecules. Membranes, 9.5 nm; ferritin, 12 nm; Fab' fragments, 6 X 3.5 nm; anti-Fe, antiferritin. Adapted from the work of A. Knüsel, T. H. Bächli, R. Gitzelmann, and J. Lindenmann, *J. Immunol.*, 106:583, 1971.

ferritin. The $F(ab')_2$ antiferritin has been purified by precipitation with ferritin and elution from immune precipitates prior to admixture with the nonpurified $F(ab')_2$ antisucrase. In contrast to the results with ferritin-*labeled* antisucrase, the hybrid antibody has localized the enzyme only at contiguous intervillar surfaces. The tips of the microvilli (Fig. 4-9) and non-contiguous villar surfaces (Fig. 4-11) are free of ferritin. Apparently, antibody or ferritin is dissociated from the tissue during immunostaining or subsequent processing. In all likelihood this dissociation is not an inherent property of the hybrid antibody, as it has been shown that Fab fragments bind specific ligands (antigen groups) with the same avidity as undigested antibody. The dissociation is not due to unusually poor binding avidity of antisucrase, because it does not occur when ferritin-labeled antisucrase is used. Furthermore, in immunocytochemistry excess of antibody is applied to tissue antigen to insure that antibodies with high avidity bind tissue antigen preferentially over those with low avidity.

Two factors, however, favor dissociation of ferritin. First, purified antiferritin has been used to make the hybrid antibody. Although purification of antiferritin often can be carried out with high yields (about 70%), it still discriminates against the strongest binding antibodies and yields preferentially those species of antibodies that have relatively weak binding affinities. Second, the hybridization of Fab' antiferritin with Fab' antisucrase is random in the sense that high binding avidity antisucrase may

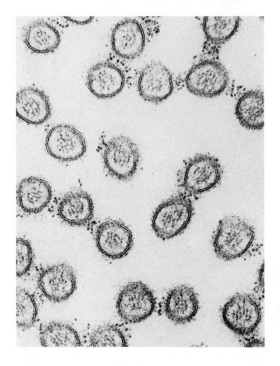

Fig. 4-11 Transverse section treated similarly as in Fig. 4-9. X90,000. Ferritin is deposited only on apposing surfaces. From A. Knüsel, T. H. Bächli, R. Gitzelmann, and J. Lindenmann, *J. Immunol.*, **106**:583, 1971.

hybridize with any antiferritin irrespective of its binding avidity. Thus, use of excess of hybrid antibody during staining while selecting high avidity antisucrase does not select high avidity antiferritin. Apparently, the combination of both factors sufficiently reduces avidity for ferritin to result in its total loss from nonapposing microvillar surfaces. One of these factors alone is probably not sufficient for dissociation, since hybrid antibody made from nonpurified antiferritin is capable of continuous localization of ferritin on a cell surface (Fig. 4-7).

Specifically localized ferritin is not lost in the space between apposing microvilli where their equidistant localization suggests multiple binding of ferritin to both microvillar surfaces (Fig. 4-10). The binding strength for ferritin increases exponentially with the number of Fab' sites reacting per molecule of ferritin.

INDIRECT STAINING WITH HYBRID ANTIBODIES

In the indirect technique cell surface antigen is first localized with unlabeled specific antiserum. This is followed by anti-IgG/anti-ferritin hybrid antibody, and ferritin, or by anti-IgG/anti-SBMV hybrid antibody, and SBMV. In the procedure for preparation of anti-IgG/antiferritin hybrid antibodies as introduced into immunocytochemistry by Hämmerling and co-workers, antiferritin is purified by specific precipitation and elution twice, once before and once after hybridization. Specific purification has not been used in the preparation of anti-IgG/anti-SBMV hybrids.

The distribution of cell surface antigen is important for differentiating origin and function of cells that are not distinguishable by morphology alone (such as different classes of lymphocytes). In the hands of Aoki and co-workers, the indirect hybrid antibody method has facilitated characterization of the apparent distribution of several antigens characteristic of circulating mouse cells. H-2 (histocompatibility) antigens occur in patches on most mouse cells. Their distribution is more abundant on thymic than on peripheral lymphoid cells (Fig. 4-12). Plasma cells and eosinophils exhibit similar amounts of H-2 antigens, while erythrocytes possess only sparse distribution (Fig. 4-13). On reticular cells, on the other hand, nearly the entire cell surface is covered by H-2 antigens, although patches of microvillar protrusions are often negative. Interestingly, peritoneal macrophages are deficient in H-2 antigen, at least on their cell surfaces.

θ antigen is not a histocompatibility antigen and is not genetically linked with the H-2 antigen. One or the other allelic forms of this antigen occurs

Fig. 4-12 Distribution of H-2, TL, and Θ alloantigens on thymus, lymph node, and spleen lymphocytes. From T. Aoki, U. Hämmerling, E. de Harven, E. A. Booyse, and L. J. Old, *J. Exp. Med.*, **130**:979, 1969.

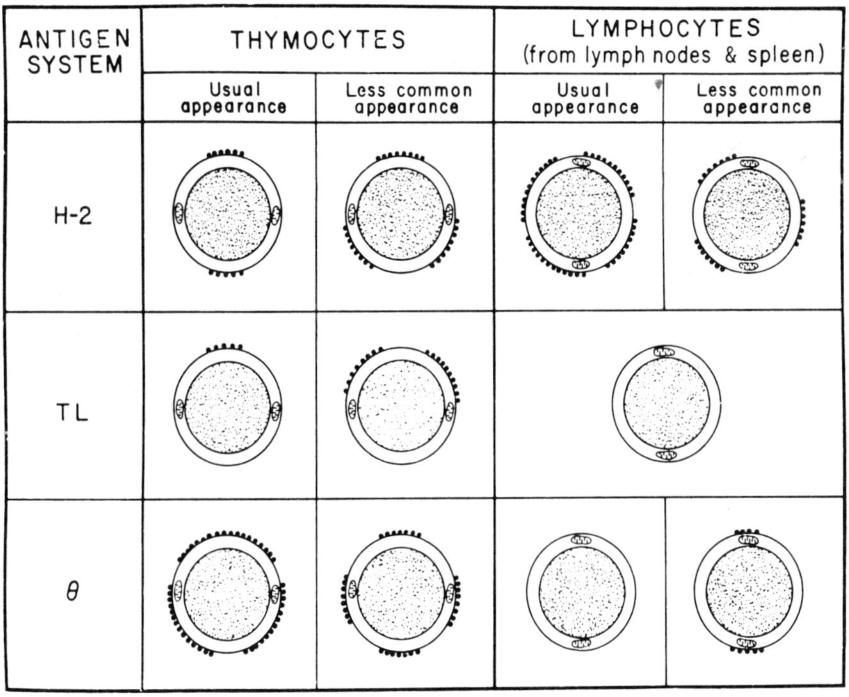

ANTIGEN SYSTEM	THYMOCYTES		LYMPHOCYTES (from lymph nodes & spleen)	
	Usual appearance	Less common appearance	Usual appearance	Less common appearance
H-2				
TL				
θ				

ERYTHROCYTE   EOSINOPHIL LEUKOCYTE   PLASMA CELL

RETICULAR CELL   PERITONEAL MACROPHAGE

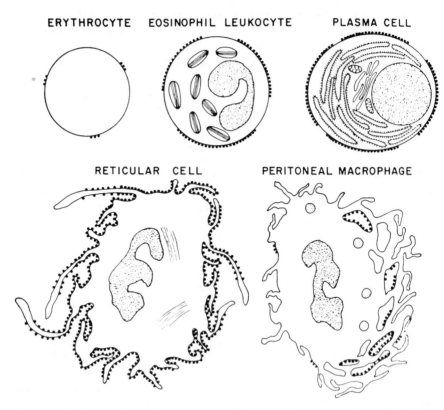

Fig. 4-13 Distribution of H-2 alloantigen on nonlymphoid cells. From T. Aoki, U. Hämmerling, E. de Harven, E. A. Booyse, and L. J. Old, *J. Exp. Med.*, **130**:979, 1969.

on all mouse thymic lymphocytes and in mouse brain. Immunocytochemically it is seen in large patches on thymic lymphocytes occupying most of the cell surface. Spleen and lymph node lymphocytes are either devoid of θ antigen or possess only small patches.

Thymus leukemia (TL) antigens are present in the genome of normal mice. They are linked to the H-2 locus. When phenotypically expressed, TL antigens are found on thymic lymphocytes only. Their distribution again is patchy.

Although the distribution of the three antigens appears as patchy on most cells, thymic lymphocytes do have an almost complete θ coat and reticular cells and peripheral lymphocytes an almost complete H-2 coat.

We have already seen that viruses that infect cells by fusion impart their envelope to part of the host cell surface. There is also evidence for exclusion of some and close association of other normal cell surface constituents from the envelope of budding progeny virus. Gross leukemia virus is a murine virus that buds from the surface of infected cells. The question whether the budding virus incorporates part of the cell surface may be answered by studies of distribution of alloantigens (such as $H2^6$, $H2^k$, θ, Ly-A, and Ly-B). In many tumor viruses, cell surface antigens are an expression of the latent viral genome. Antisera to these antigens fail to neutralize the virus. The question whether the Gross leukemia genome on infection of mouse cells specifies elements of the cell surface other than those comprising viral envelopes may be answered by studying in histocompatible mouse strains the cellular distribution of antigens reactive with antisera to Gross leukemia. These antisera are cytotoxic but do not neutralize Gross leukemia virus. They are exceptional as most other RNA leukemia virus antisera contain cytotoxic, as well as antiviral antibodies. Application of Gross antiserum to leukemia cells followed by the indirect hybrid antibody—ferritin or SBMV technique, indeed, reveals a patchy distribution of the antigen on the cell surface. The virions (virus particles with capsules as viewed in the electron microscope) are free of antigen (Figs. 4-2 and 4-3). Application of H-2, Ly-A, or Ly-B antiserum followed by the hybrid antibody method again reveals patchy distribution of histocompatibility antigens on the cell surface, and again the budding virions are free of antigen. Therefore, neither the major normal host cell antigens nor the Gross virus-specified cellular antigens are part of the Gross virion.

Occasional virions do, however, bear θ or $H\text{-}2^k$ antigens on parts of their surfaces when budding from cells possessing these alloantigens. The fractions of total virus and cell surfaces that are labeled are approximately equal. Apparently, the presence of θ or $H\text{-}2^k$ antigen on a cell membrane segment neither restricts nor promotes the budding of the virus from it. In contrast budding of virus is excluded from segments that bear $H\text{-}2^b$, Ly-A, or Ly-B alloantigens, or Gross leukemia envelope antigen. Interestingly, the $H\text{-}2^k$ allele confers sensitivity and the $H\text{-}2^b$ allele resistance to spontaneous Gross leukemia in mice.

THE QUESTION OF PATCHY DISTRIBUTION OF ANTIGENS ON LIVING CELL SURFACES

Cells in suspension culture continually extend and retract pseudopods and continually imbibe surrounding medium into newly formed vacuoles. Protein assembly on polysomal membranes is rapid. The half-life of messenger RNA is short. Cellular events suggest that the membranes that channel them are continually changing. It is probable, therefore, that in a living cell individual antigen sites are not static as seen in electron microscopic immunocytochemistry. While the membrane may serve to confine the antigen to a surface and prevent its solubilization by cell sap or extracellular fluid, it is likely that antigen is subject to continuous motion on the cell surface, such as bubbles on the surface of water. Without such continuous motion, the flexibility and changeability of cellular membranes would be difficult to conceive. Application of antibody to a living cell when it results in specific binding with a constituent of the cell membrane does not in itself immobilize a cell membrane antigen. By the time we have completed a cytochemical procedure on an unfixed cell, there has been ample opportunity for cell surface antigens to rearrange. Hence, we may ask to what extent does an observed patchy immunocytochemical distribution of antigen on the cell surface reflect the true situation prior to staining?

The question is important because much work in electron immunocytochemistry is done with cell surface antigens, and often special effort is made to stain a viable cell. In most instances immunocytochemical observations have revealed discontinuous distribution of cell surface antigens. The distribution of antigens on erythrocytes appears to follow a fairly well defined periodicity when stained by the indirect ferritin-labeled antibody method. Similarly, alloantigens on lymphoid cells yield patchy distribution either by the indirect ferritin-labeled or the indirect hybrid antibody method. The first event in an immune response is the recognition of an antigenic determinant by a specific lymphoid cell possessing the proper receptor. In search for the immediately ensuing events after recognition, much significance is being attributed to the rearrangement of distribution of the recognizing unit after combination with antigen (page 200). To insure useful interpretation of these observations, it is important to understand to what extent immunocytochemical observations reflect true antigen distribution prior to staining.

W. C. Davis has been the first to note that the patchy distribution of alloantigens on cell surfaces may be a staining artifact. On application of H-2 alloantiserum to mouse lymphocytes followed by ferritin-labeled anti-IgG, the distribution of antigen occurs in widely separated patches (Fig. 4-14). However, when immunoglobulin from the same alloantiserum is

Fig. 4-14 Patchy localization of H-2 antigen on B-10A lymphocytes by B-10M serum anti-B 10A spleen cells followed by ferritin-conjugated rabbit immunoglobulin antimouse IgG. X67,250. From W. C. Davis, M. A. Alspaugh, J. H. Stimpfling, and R. L. Walford, *Tissue Antigens*, 1:89, 1971.

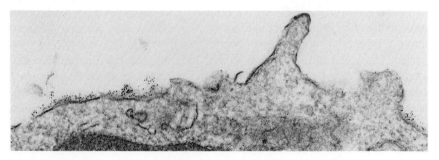

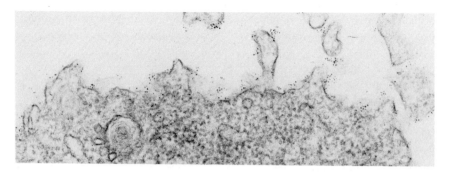

Fig. 4-15 Largely continuous localization of H-2 antigen on B10A lymphocytes by ferritin-conjugated B10M immunoglobulin anti-B10A spleen cells. X67,250. From W. C. Davis, M. A. Alspaugh, J. H. Stimpfling, and R. C. Walford, *Tissue Antigens,* 1:89, 1971.

conjugated with ferritin and used in the direct technique, the distribution becomes continuous (Fig. 4-15). This continuous localization can be reverted to patchy localization if application of the ferritin-labeled alloantibody is followed either by unlabeled antiferritin or unlabeled antimouse immunoglobulin. The data permit the conclusion that patchy distribution is an artifact of the indirect ferritin-labeled antibody technique. Ferritin-labeled anti-IgG usually consists of ferritin-conjugated antibody that is largely monovalent and nonagglutinating (page 65) plus a small amount of unconjugated antibody that is divalent (page 62). It is apparently the divalent antibody that aggregates the anti-H2 into patches. This aggregation seems to be facilitated by the lack of a fixed position of H-2 antigen on the cell membrane. In the direct ferritin-labeled antibody technique, the aggregation does not occur, apparently because the ferritin-labeled antibody is largely monovalent and because the small amount of contaminating unconjugated bivalent antibody is probably insufficient in concentration. Nevertheless, even in the direct technique the distribution is not entirely uniform (Fig. 4-14). In the indirect technique aggregation is probably caused by the cooperative effect of a small amount of contaminating, unlabeled bivalent anti-IgG and the large amount of bivalent unlabeled anti-H2. (This is reminiscent of the failure of spontaneous agglutination of cells obtained from the circulation of patients with autoimmune hemolytic anemia and their agglutination *in vitro* once anti-immunoglobulin is added.)

The findings of Davis also explain the patchy distribution of allo-antigens and Gross leukemia antigens with hybrid anti-SBMV employed in indirect technique The hybrid antibody is monovalent with regard to each of its functions and, therefore, cannot cross-link two mouse immunoglobulin molecules. However in the preparation of the hybrid antibody, the antiimmunoglobulin/antiimmunoglobulin recombinants have not been separated (page 101). The Three factors may, therefore, contribute to conglutination of antigen sites into patches: bivalent, unlabeled anticell surface antibody, contaminating anti-IgG/anti-IgG recombinants, and multiplicity of identical antigen sites on the SBMV surface that permits simultaneous binding with several hybrid antibody molecules (Fig. 4-16).

When anti-IgG/antiferritin is used in the indirect hybrid antibody method, usually the antiferritin is immunospecifically separated from anti-IgG/anti-IgG recombinants. This eliminates an important factor for aggregation of surface-bound IgG. Nevertheless, distribution of surface antigens is patchy. Indeed, the method still incorporates two factors that could cause aggregation of antigen into patches: the unlabeled anticell surface antibody and multiple attachment of a ferritin molecule to several hybrid antibodies (Fig. 4-17). However, even if only a fraction of the cell antigens is conglutinated, it would probably only be the conglutinated patches that come under electron microscopic visualization. The ferritin on nonconglutinated parts of the surface would be attached to a single hybrid antibody molecule only. The ferritin-hybrid antibody bond is easily dissociated since the hybrid antibody has been specifically purified, as we have seen in the case of localization of intestinal sucrase (page 99). In the conglutinated patches, on the other hand, ferritin is held by multiple bonding. Hence, it is dissociated with much greater difficulty. Thus, only the conglutinated patches would come to electron microscopic observation.

The redistribution of surface antigens during staining may be averted by fixation of the cell, or, perhaps, by treatment with sodium azide, or nitrophenol. Alternatively one may, perhaps, substitute Fab for antibody in the first and second step of the indirect ferritin-labeled antibody technique.

The patchy distribution of cell-surface antigens has only been observed with indirect techniques using autoimmune or alloantisera. These antisera usually are not very rich in antibody contents and, hence, it is difficult to achieve antibody excess. We may expect, therefore, that the antibodies are bound to the cell surface via both their specific combining sites. The bivalent binding of antibody to surface antigen molecules bearing multiple antigen sites predisposes to aggregation into patches. With heteroimmune antisera large amounts of antibodies are usually produced, and one may expect that if these sera are used in excess only one of the combining sites of their antibodies reacts with cell-surface antigen determinants, while the other binding site remains free. In an indirect technique conglutination of surface antigen would be averted if the second antibody is largely monovalent or if a bivalent second antibody would be applied in high excess. Continuous localization has, indeed, been observed on mouse plasmacytoma cells stained with undiluted rat serum antimouse plasmacytoma followed by

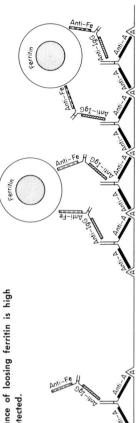

Fig. 4-16 (At left.) Presumptive mechanism of patch formation in localization of surface antigens on unfixed cells by the indirect anti-IgG/anti-SBMV hybrid antibody technique. Co-operative effect of the unlabeled anticell antibody, contaminating anti-IgG/anti-IgG recom-binants and multivalence of southern bean mosaic virus (SBMV). Seven antigen sites (A) are conglutinated by 4 anti-A molecules, one anti-IgG/anti-IgG recombinant, and one SBMV particle.

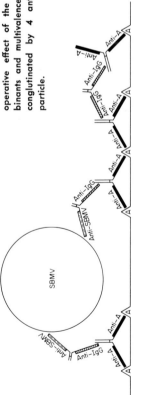

Fig. 4-17 (Below.) Presumptive mechanism of patch formation in staining of surface antigens on unfixed cells by the indirect anti-IgG/antiferritin hybrid antibody technique. The hybrid antibody is freed of anti-IgG/anti-IgG recombinants. Aggregation of the cell antigen (A) into patches is the cooperative result of the unlabeled anti-A and the multivalency of ferritin. Be-cause of the absence of bivalent anti-IgG, patch formation in the present situation is expected to be less than in Fig. 4-16. The patches envisaged are shown on the right side. Some antigen sites may well remain nonconglutinated as illustrated on the left side. However, the anti-IgG/antiferritin is of low binding avidity for ferritin, and the chance of loosing ferritin is high (see text). Hence, nonconglutinated sites may remain largely undetected.

a largely univalent labeled antibody conjugate (Chapter 5). Localization is also continuous on sheep erythrocytes treated with undiluted rabbit anti-erythrocyte serum; sheep erythrocytes reacted with the third component of complement (C3), and treated with rabbit anti-C3; and on thrombocytes treated with rabbit antithrombosthenin, followed in each case with an excess of unlabeled bivalent sheep serum antirabbit IgG (pages 154, 157, and 173).

The hybrid antibody method avoids nonspecificity as it uses unlabeled antibodies only. In the direct application the ideal of depositing a single detector molecule (ferritin) to a single antigen site can be approached. To utilize all the potential of the method, it appears desirable to find a procedure that insures inclusion of only avid antiferritin in the hybrid antibody and exclusion at the same time of interfering recombinants.

REFERENCES

Aoki, T., Boyse, E. A., Old, L. J., de Harven, E., Hämmerling, U., and Wood, H. A. G(Gross) and H-2 cell-surface antigens: Location on Gross leukemia cells by electron microscopy with visually labeled antibody. *Proc. Natl. Acad. Sci., U.S.,* **65**:569, 1970.

Aoki, T., Hämmerling, U., de Harven, E., Boyse, E. A., and Old, L. J. Antigenic structure of cell surfaces. An immunoferritin study of the occurrence and topography of H-2, θ, and TL alloantigens on mouse cells. *J. Exp. Med.,* **130**:979, 1969.

Aoki, T. and Takahashi, T. Viral and cellular surface antigens of murine leukemis and myelomas. *J. Exp. Med.,* **135**:443, 1972.

Davis, W. C. H-2 antigen on cell membranes: An explanation for the alteration of distribution by indirect labeling techniques. *Science,* **175**:1006, 1972.

Davis, W. C., Alspaugh, M. A., Stimpfling, J. H., and Walford, R. M. Cellular surface distribution of transplantation antigens: Discrepancy between direct and indirect labeling techniques. *Tissue Antigens,* **1**:89, 1971.

Gitzelmann, R., Bächli, T. L., Binz, H., Lindenmann, J., and Semenza, G. Localization of rabbit intestinal sucrase with ferritin-antibody conjugates. *Biochim. Biophys. Acta,* **196**:20, 1970.

Hämmerling, U., Aoki, T., de Harven, E., Boyse, E. A., and Old, L. J. Use of hybrid antibody with anti-IgG and antiferritin specificities in locating cell surface antigens by electron microscopy. *J. Exp. Med.,* **128**:1461, 1968.

Hämmerling, U., Aoki, T., Wood, H. A., Boyse, E. A., and de Harven, E. New visual markers of antibody for electron microscopy. *Nature,* **223**:1158, 1969.

Heine, J. W. and Schnaitman, C. A. Entry of vesicular stomatitis virus into L-cells. *J. Virol.,* **8**:786, 1971.

Knüsel, A., Bächli, T. L., Gitzelmann, R., and Lindenmann, J. Electron microscopic recognition of surface antigen by direct reaction and ferritin capture with guinea pig hybrid antibody. *J. Immunol.,* **106**:583, 1971.

Wagner, R. R., Heine, J. W., Goldstein, G., and Schnaitman, C. A. Use of antiviral-antiferritin hybrid antibody for localization of viral antigen in plasma membrane. *J. Virol.,* **7**:274, 1971.

Chapter 5

Enzyme-Conjugated
Antibody Methods

Enzymes have for long been demonstrated cytochemically. Substrate selectivity is the key to the specificity of their localization. Catalytic production of a large number of product molecules is the basis of the sensitivity of their localization. The requirements for successful cytochemical demonstration of enzymes by light and electron microscopy include availability of a soluble substrate that forms upon enzyme action, a product that can either be precipitated by a capturing agent, or can undergo secondary precipitation spontaneously. If the precipitate itself is not colored or electron-opaque, these properties may be conferred upon it in a separate step. For electron microscopic enzyme cytochemistry, precipitation must be exceedingly rapid; otherwise, diffusion prior to precipitation distorts resolution. As suggested in a review by T. K. Shnitka and A. M. Seligman, the addition of an extrinsic capturing agent for precipitation of the product (via salt formation, a secondary organic reaction, or addition of a secondary enzyme system) may not always give optimal resolution, because either the product is too soluble, or crystalline (such as most salts), or the precipitation too slow relative to the diffusion of the enzyme product from its site of formation. Hence, the best resolutions have been obtained with products that precipitate spontaneously and are amorphous. The lowest solubilities and the most amorphous end products have been obtained with polymers. The cytochemical demonstration of peroxidase provides an example. The substrate for peroxidase is hydrogen peroxide. Enzyme action does not continue in the absence of an electron donor. The electron donor is oxidized at the very site of action of the enzyme and not at a distance from it. Diaminobenzidine (Fig. 5-1), when donating electrons to hydrogen peroxide via peroxidase, apparently forms an oxidative intermediate that rapidly polymerizes to an amorphous, insoluble, brown deposit suitable for light microscopy. Added osmium tetroxide is rapidly reduced and chelated by this polymer, leading to precipitation at the site of enzyme action of a black,

110

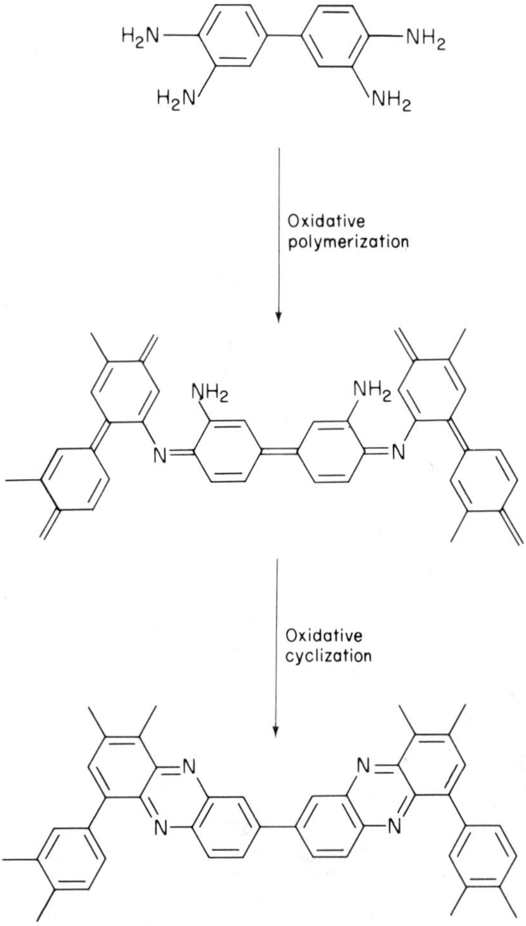

Fig. 5-1 Peroxidase donates electrons to hydrogen peroxide. The oxidized enzyme is reconstituted to the reduced form by an electron donor, such as diaminobenzidine. The free bonds of the oxidation product of diaminobenzidine rapidly react with each other to form an insoluble phenazine polymer of somewhat hypothetical composition. The polymer forms a highly insoluble, amorphous, electron-opaque chelate with osmium tetroxide deposited at the site of enzyme action. From A. M. Seligman and co-workers, *J. Cell Biol.*, **38**:1, 1972.

electron-opaque, insoluble, low valence, chelated product of osmium. For this reason enzymes that rapidly accept electrons from diaminobenzidine are eminently suitable for histochemical detection by light and electron microscopy.

Another example of cytochemical detection of an enzyme via formation of a polymer is the light and electron microscopic detection of acetylcholinesterase. The enzyme hydrolyzes acetate from many esters, some of which provide suitable cytochemical substrates such as the thioester shown in Fig. 5-2. Enzyme action liberates the thiol that rapidly reacts with the diazonium group, forming diazothioether polymers that are visualized by reduction of osmium tetroxide.

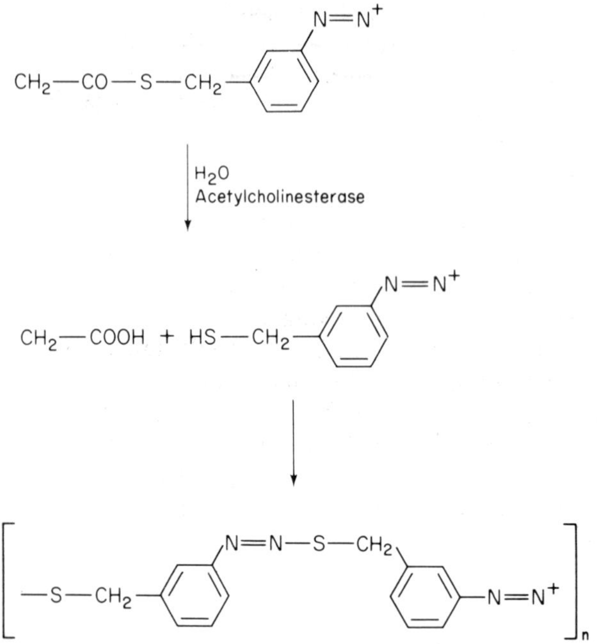

Fig. 5-2 Another example of enzyme cytochemistry via polymer formation. Acetylcholinesterase action frees a thiol group and converts, thereby, a monofunctional substance (diazonium) to a bifunctional substance (diazonium plus thiol). Both functional groups interact, forming linear diazothioether polymers that are osmiophilic.

The ease of cytochemical visualization of enzymes can be utilized in immunocytochemistry, provided the enzyme is attached specifically to a tissue antigen site. One means of accomplishing this is by chemical conjugation of the enzyme to specific antibodies using procedures that resemble, in many ways, those we have seen in the ferritin-conjugated antibody method. We have reason to believe that, at least in theory, such procedure affords an enzymatic, cytochemical intensification of the antigen-antibody reaction. Indeed, we are from the very onset somewhat better off than the enzyme cytochemist. While the enzyme cytochemist must find a suitable substrate for the very enzyme he investigates, we can, in immunocytochemistry. choose among many enzymes those most suitable for our purpose. We would like to use the following criteria in our choice:

1. The enzyme should be easily detectable by a cytochemical method, preferably one applicable to light and electron microscopy. To insure high resolution the enzyme-reaction product should not diffuse away from the production site. The cytochemical substrate should have a high turnover number with the enzyme in neutral buffers that do not affect tissue structure severely.

2. The enzyme should be available in pure form.

3. Conjugation with immunoglobulin should not abolish enzyme activity, although it may impair it.

4. The enzyme should be fairly stable in neutral solution.

5. Preferably, the enzyme should be of relatively small molecular weight, as small enzyme-antibody complexes penetrate tissue somewhat better than larger complexes.

6. Preferably, substrate-related enzymes should not be found as endogenous constituents of the tissues examined.

Horseradish peroxidase fulfills these criteria best. The diaminobenzidine-hydrogen peroxide method of Graham and Karnovsky is one of the best light and electron microscopic cytochemical methods available. In horseradishes the substance responsible for the tear-promoting effect, an allylisocyanate, reacts with peroxidase and blocks most of its available amino groups. For conjugation with immunoglobulin, bifunctional amino acid reagents are used. R. R. Modesto and A. J. Pesce have shown that not more than 1.7 amino groups per molecule are available for this binding, even when excess bifunctional reagent is used. The limited extent of reaction assures that enzyme activity is not reduced as a result of exposure to conjugating agent.

One-Step Conjugation of Peroxidase with Immunoglobulin: Principle

4,4'-difluoro-3,3'-dinitrodiphenyl sulfone (FNPS) has been introduced by P. K. Nakane and G. B. Pierce and glutaraldehyde by S. Avrameas for the cross-linking of peroxidase to immunoglobulin (Fig. 5-3). In the FNPS procedure 0.2 μM of immunoglobulin are admixed with 1.25 μM of peroxidase and 36 μM of FNPS. In the glutaraldehyde procedure 0.32 μM of immunoglobulin or purified antibody are admixed with 3 μM of peroxidase and 5 μM of glutaraldehyde. It has been shown by Modesto and Pesce, using FNPS, that reaction with IgG is 66 times faster than with peroxidase. Thus, if an IgG molecule has reacted with one or more FNPS groups (or presumably glutaraldehyde groups), it has a 66 fold greater chance to cross-link with another IgG molecule than with a peroxidase molecule. Consequently, the predominant reaction products are polymers of immunoglobulin that are either devoid of peroxidase or contain, occasionally, one peroxidase molecule. No polymers of peroxidase form. Only 1% of total peroxidase enters the conjugate. The remainder is lost (Fig. 5-4). When using the above-mentioned proportions of FNPS and proteins, peroxidase in the isolated conjugate fraction contains on the average 0.682, and IgG, 1.3 FNPS groups per molecule. In these proportions the amount of available FNPS is limited, and formation of large polymers of IgG (Fig. 5-4, peak 1) is kept to a minimum, while a large excess of

$$F-\overset{NO_2}{\underset{}{C_6H_3}}-\overset{O}{\underset{O}{S}}-\overset{NO_2}{\underset{}{C_6H_3}}-F \xrightarrow{\text{protein}-NH_2} \text{protein}-NH-\overset{NO_2}{\underset{}{C_6H_3}}-\overset{O}{\underset{O}{S}}-\overset{NO_2}{\underset{}{C_6H_3}}-NH-\text{protein}$$

$$\overset{O}{\underset{H}{C}}-CH_2-CH_2-CH_2-\overset{O}{\underset{H}{C}} \xrightarrow{\text{protein}-NH_2} \text{protein}-N=CH-CH_2-CH_2-CH_2-CH=N-\text{protein}$$

Fig. 5-3 4,4′-difluoro-3,3′-dinitrodiphenyl sulfone (FNPS) or glutaraldehyde are commonly employed bifunctional reagents to cross-link two protein molecules or to polymerize them. Both react with available amino groups in protein (ϵ-amino groups of lysine and N-terminal amino groups). Because of a large number of available amino groups in immunoglobulin and an abnormally small number in peroxidase (1.7 per molecule on the average), reaction with immunoglobulin is 66 times faster than with peroxidase. Consequently, homologous reaction between two immunoglobulin molecules is preferred over heterologous reaction of immunoglobulin with peroxidase. Upon extensive reaction the multivalency of available amino groups in immunoglobulin and most other proteins favors formation of large aggregates and precipitation. The limited number of available amino groups in peroxidase precludes homopolymerization, precipitation, or inactivation of peroxidase. Glutaraldehyde is water soluble, but FNPS possesses low solubility under the conditions of conjugation of peroxidase with immunoglobulin commonly employed (single-step addition at low temperature). Consequently, conjugation of FNPS and immunoglobulin tends to be incomplete, leaving the bulk of immunoglobulin unconjugated. The mildness of the procedure precludes excessive formation of polymeric immunoglobulin. Conjugation with glutaraldehyde tends to react all available immunoglobulin, and polymeric immunoglobulin forms. FNPS reacts more completely if added to the reaction mixture at 37° in repeated small batches and if pH 10.5 is maintained during the entire course of the reaction. In the case of FNPS, hydrolysis competes with protein aminolysis. In order to promote the reaction with protein amine, conjugation must be carried out at high pH. Hydrolysis precludes retention of unreacted fluoronitrobenzene in the conjugate. In the case of glutaraldehyde, reaction with water is no major problem. In fact precautions must be taken against nonspecific reaction of conjugate with tissue amine because of retention of unreacted aldehyde groups (glutaraldehyde in which only one aldehyde group has reacted with protein, while the other aldehyde group remains free). Free aldehyde groups can be destroyed by lysine, or if after conjugation Tris buffer is used as solvent and if the conjugate is stored prior to use. Other side reactions of conjugation are intramolecular bonding of *both* active groups of the bifunctional reagent. This bonding is often preferred over the intermolecular reaction.

Fig. 5-4 Gel filtration (Sephadex G-200, 0.1 M phosphate buffer, pH 7.0, 4°) of peroxidase-immunoglobulin conjugate made with 4,4′-difluoro-3,3′-dinitrodiphenyl sulfone (FNPS) in a one-step reaction mixture. Input: conjugate prepared by reaction of 10 mg of peroxidase and 10 mg of goat immunoglobulin antirabbit IgG with 0.25 mg FNPS in a final volume of 0.5 ml at pH 10.0. Abscissa represents fraction number. ——— absorbance at 280 nm; ————, peroxidase activity. Peak 1 (void volume) represents polymeric immunoglobulin. Peak 2 represents unconjugated immunoglobulin. Peak 3 represents unconjugated peroxidase. Less than 1% of the peroxidase activity is in the major protein peak. Conjugate consisting of one molecule of peroxidase and one molecule of immunoglobulin is expected to elute in the poorly separated zone between peaks 1 and 2. From R. R. Modesto and A. G. Pesce, *Biophys. Biochem. Acta,* **229:**384, 1971.

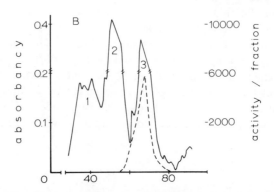

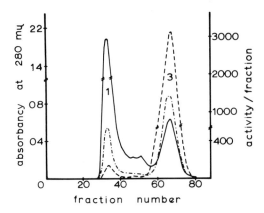

Fig. 5-5 Gel filtration (Sephadex G-200, 0.2 M carbonate buffer, pH 10.0, 4°) of peroxidase-immunoglobulin conjugate made by separate additions of FNPS to a one-step reaction mixture. Input: conjugate prepared by reaction of a mixture of 18.7 mg peroxidase and 10 mg IgG with six additions of a total of 19.13 mg FNPS in a final volume of 2.4 ml at constantly maintained a pH 10.5 at room temperature for three hours. ————, absorbance at 280 nm; — • —, absorbance at 403 nm; ———, peroxidase activity. Peak 1 (void volume) represents polymeric IgG. Peak 3 represents unconjugated peroxidase. Little protein elutes in a position corresponding to unconjugated immunoglobulin (about fraction number 50). 4.5% of the peroxidase activity elutes with peak 1. From R. R. Modesto and A. J. Pesce, *Biophys. Biochem. Acta*, **229**:384, 1971.

unconjugated immunoglobulin is retained (peak 2). The small amount of peroxidase activity that is eluted under peaks 1 and 2 is difficult to separate from the excess of monomeric and polymeric immunoglobulin devoid of peroxidase. The unconjugated immunoglobulin competes with conjugate for antigen sites and reduces efficiency of staining.

If conditions of reaction are changed by increasing the ratio of peroxidase to IgG, increasing the amount of FNPS, carrying out conjugation at 25° instead of 4°, and adding FNPS gradually while maintaining the pH at 10.5, nearly all the IgG becomes polymeric (Fig. 5-5, peak 1), unreacted IgG almost disappears, and most peroxidase still remains monomeric (peak 3).

Similar conditions prevail in the cross-linking of peroxidase and immunoglobulin with glutaraldehyde. On ultracentrifugation of the conjugate prepared with glutaraldehyde at the proportions given above (page 113), the only discernible peak is due to unconjugated peroxidase. The IgG peak has disappeared and is replaced by polydisperse material unable to produce a Schlieren boundary. This indicates that the original IgG has been transformed to polymers of IgG of varying sizes. These polymers contain either no peroxidase or rarely more than one molecule. If immunoglobulin

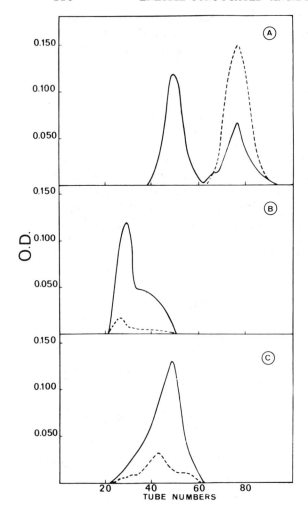

Fig. 5-6 Gel filtration (Sephadex G-200, 0.1 M phosphate buffer, pH 6.8) of peroxidase-immunoglobulin conjugate prepared with glutaraldehyde. A, standardization of column with mixture of purified sheep anti-rabbit IgG and peroxidase. B, conjugate prepared by single-step procedure and separated from free peroxidase by ammonium sulfate precipitation. Nearly all protein elutes with the void volume, indicating polymerization. C, conjugate prepared by two-step procedure. Most of the antibody (solid line peak) remains unconjugated. Most of the conjugated peroxidase (broken line peak) elutes after the void volume, indicating complexes of one peroxidase with one antibody molecule. Solid line, absorbence at 280 nm. Broken line, absorbence at 403 nm. From S. Avrameas, *Immunochemistry*, 8:1175 1971.

and conjugate are separated from free peroxidase by half saturation with ammonium sulfate, the redissolved precipitate passes through a Sephadex G 200-column with the void volume (Fig. 5-6B). Again no unconjugated immunoglobulin is present. In conjugate so prepared by S. Avrameas and B. Guilbert with purified antibody, the peroxidase antibody ratio was 1:3, and since no unconjugated, unpolymerized antibody was present one must assume that on the average the conjugate consisted of trimers of immuno-globulin bound with a single molecule of peroxidase. If prepared from anti-IgG, preservation of antibody activity was 85%. If prepared from anti-tyrosinase or antilactate dehydrogenase, less than 5% of antibody activity was preserved. Since purified anti-IgG was used, six specific antibody combining sites contributed to one trimeric molecule. Thus, 85% retention of antibody activity indicates that in 15% of conjugated molecules all the six combining sites have been hindered. The chance of hindrance of a single site as a result of conjugation in anti-IgG is, therefore, $\sqrt[6]{0.15} = 73\%$. The chance of hindrance of a single site in the antityrosinase or antilactate dehydrogenase is more than $\sqrt[6]{0.95} = 99\%$.

If instead of purified antibodies we were to conjugate IgG and assuming the IgG is from a hyperimmune serum so that as much as $\frac{1}{6}$ of all the IgG is specific antibody, then 58% of the trimers would contain only nonspecific IgG, and 35% would contain one, 7% two, and only a negligible fraction three specific antibody molecules. In the case of anti-IgG, the chance of loss of all antibody activity in the IgG trimer containing one specific antibody molecule is $(0.73)^2 = 53\%$ and in the trimers containing two specific molecules $(0.73)^4 = 28\%$. The fraction of trimers retaining at least one specific antibody site is, therefore $[0.35 \cdot (1 - 0.53) + 0.07 \cdot (1 - 0.28)] = 22\%$. In the case of the antityrosinase and antilactate dehydrogenase, the chance of loss of all antibody activity in the IgG trimers containing one specific antibody molecule is more than $(0.99)^2 = 98\%$ and in the trimeric IgG containing two specific antibody molecules more than $(0.99)^4 = 96\%$. The fraction of trimers retaining at least one specific antibody site will, therefore, be less than $[0.35 \cdot (1 - 0.98) + 0.07 \cdot (1 - 0.96)] = 1\%$.

These considerations show that if in conjugation IgG is used instead of purified antibody the retention of antibody binding activity is reduced. Of course, a conjugate molecule contains only 3 IgG and 1 PO subunit on the average. Some complexes are smaller, and others are larger. Chances are greater for the larger immunoglobulin aggregates to contain any peroxidase than for the smaller ones. The smaller complexes penetrate tissue faster than the larger ones and arrive at specific sites earlier, thus, exacerbating the competition with peroxidase-conjugated antibody for specific antigen sites.

In summary, analysis of conjugates of peroxidase with immunoglobulin indicates that:

1. Peroxidase activity is not lost during conjugation. The enzymatic amplification for a specifically localized conjugate molecule is high.

2. It is the efficiency of immunohistochemical localization that is low and impairs the overall sensitivity. Efficiency is lowered because of losses of peroxidase during conjugation, extensive destruction of antibody activity if immunoglobulin rather than purified antibody is used, and moderate to extensive competition for conjugate by native or polymerized unconjugated immunoglobulin.

ONE-STEP CONJUGATION OF PEROXIDASE WITH IMMUNOGLOBULIN: PROCEDURE

In the procedure of S. Avrameas, 0.05 ml of a 1% aqueous solution of glutaraldehyde are added slowly under gentle stirring to 5 mg of purified antibody and 10 mg of peroxidase dissolved in 1.0 ml of 0.1 M phosphate buffer, pH 6.8. After two hours standing at room temperature, the solution is dialyzed against buffered saline at 4° overnight. A precipitate is removed in a Spinco rotor 40 at 20,000 rpm at 4°. Conjugate may be separated from peroxidase by addition of an equal volume of saturated ammonium sulfate solution, washing the precipitate twice in half-saturated ammonium sulfate solution, dissolving it in a small volume of water, and dialyzing the solution against Tris buffer or against lysine-containing phosphate buffer at 4° for one week.

ONE-STEP PREPARED CONJUGATES OF PEROXIDASE AND IMMUNOGLOBULIN: STAINING

Direct or indirect technique can be used. For light microscopy, tissue preparation and incubation times resemble those of immunofluorescence. Peroxidase is detected by incubation in 0.05% diaminobenzidine tetrahydrochloride and 0.001–0.01% hydrogen peroxidase in 0.05 M Tris buffer, pH 7.6, for 5–30 minutes. Sections can be observed with or without postosmication.

In staining tissue for electron microscopy prior to embedding, long incubation times are needed to obtain optimal penetration of conjugate. Washing times must also be prolonged. Since prolonged exposure to hydrogen peroxide is damaging to tissue and since diaminobenzidine penetrates tissues somewhat slower than hydrogen peroxide, the enzyme reaction is sometimes developed by prolonged incubation in diaminobenzidine followed by addition of hydrogen peroxide during the last half hour only. Osmication is necessary to confer electron opacity to the reaction product. Because of the effects of fixatives on antigenic reactivity and on permeability of tissues to antibodies, tissues are rarely fixed optimally prior to completion of reaction with antibody. Since peroxidase activity itself is not affected by glutaraldehyde, refixation in 4% glutaraldehyde for 20 minutes after application of conjugate and washing is desirable. Diaminobenzidine and hydrogen peroxide are applied after removal of the fixative by further washing. The glutaraldehyde protects tissue against damage by hydrogen peroxide. Addition of 0.5 M sucrose to all fixatives is also important to stabilize tissue structure.

One of the finest demonstrations of electron microscopic staining with peroxidase-conjugated antibodies is the localization of collagen on tendons of the dermis in newborn and adult chickens reported by Livia Lustig (Fig. 5.7). Following fixation in 4% depolymerized paraformaldehyde for four hours at 4°, 30 μ thick cryostat sections were incubated for 24 hours at 4° with peroxidase-conjugated immunoglobulin anticollagen (neutral salt-soluble collagen from chicken leg tendons). After 24 hours washing in phosphate-buffered saline, the sections were fixed in 5% buffered glutar-aldehyde, washed in phosphate-buffered saline overnight, stained with diam-inobenzidine and hydrogen peroxide, treated with 1% osmium tetroxide, dehydrated and embedded.

Staining was intense in the collagen fibers of tendons of newborn and adult chickens. The fibroblasts of adult chickens were not in active synthesis of collagen as judged from the immunocytochemical reaction. However, in young chickens some of the fibroblasts had positive staining in the dilated cisternae of the endoplasmic reticulum.

One of the most significant contributions of the enzyme-conjugated antibody method is Paul Nakane's classification of the cells of the anterior pituitary by identification of the specific hormones secreted. Several hormones can be identified on the same section in light microscopy when different substrates for peroxidase are used, each producing a deposit of different color. Thus, the gonadotropic cell is localized by application of antigonadotropin and peroxidase-conjugated anti-IgG and staining of perox-idase with 4-chloro-1-naphthol and hydrogen peroxide, forming a blue

Fig. 5-7 Dermis of newborn chicken treated with peroxidase conjugated immunoglobulin anti-collagen, counterstained with uranyl acetate. The reaction product is over the collagen fibers. X21,000. From Livia Lustig, *J. Histochem. Cytochem.*, **19:**663, 1971.

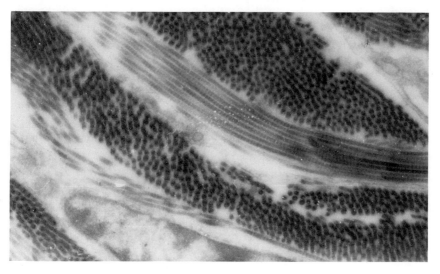

deposit. Acidification removes the antibodies from the section (page 14) but leaves the deposit unaffected. Now, corticotropin can be localized in the same section by application of anticorticotropin and, again, peroxidase-conjugated anti-IgG, followed by staining for peroxidase with diaminobenzidine and hydrogen peroxide, yielding a brown deposit.

Pituitary hormones can be directly stained on the ultrathin methacrylate or epon section. Employing indirect techniques, the sections are mildly etched and pretreated with normal serum from the species donating the conjugate in procedures resembling those used in the immunouranium and the unlabeled antibody enzyme technique (pages 57 and 158). Nakane discovered that it is important to apply the solution containing hydrogen peroxide and diaminobenzidine or chloronaphthol under continuous agitation in order to avoid build-up of large, nonspecific deposits. A 0.005% solution of diaminobenzidine tetrahydrochloride or a saturated solution of chloronaphthol containing 0.001% hydrogen peroxide is recommended. The intensity of the reaction product of chloronaphthol and hydrogen peroxide can, apparently, be enhanced by a 1% solution of copper sulfate. The secretion granules of the normal growth hormone cell, prolactin, corticotropin, and gonadotropin cell reveal several electron-opaque deposits after reaction with specific antiserum and enzyme conjugated anti-IgG. The failure of complete coverage of the granules by reaction product has been ascribed to destruction of antigen reactivity during fixation. However, complete coverage of the corticotropin secretion granules is obtained by a different method (page 161). Specific reaction product is also found at times in the cisternae of the endoplasmic reticulum and in the Golgi apparatus of the anterior lobe cells producing the four hormones.

The peroxidase-conjugated antibody method suggests that corticotropin, thyroid-stimulating hormone, and prolactin each are secreted by their own cell type. The proposed location of follicle-stimulating and luteinizing hormones in the same oval shaped cell has been confirmed with the unlabeled antibody enzyme method (Chapter 6) in the light microscopic studies of Phifer, Midgley, and Spicer, and at least the frequent association of both hormones in the same secretion granule in the electron-microscopic studies of Sternberger and Petrali.

Hypothyroidism or thyroidectomy cause a rise in the level of circulating thyrotropic hormone. Pituitary hormone levels decline, apparently, because of accelerated secretory activity of the thyrotropic cell. A hypertrophic cell, called thyroidectomy cell, can be morphologically identified by its vacuolated appearance in the anterior lobe of the pituitary. The work of Baker and Yu with peroxidase-conjugated antibody reveals extensive loss, though not entire disappearance of staining for thyrotropic hormone in the peripheral vacuolar cytoplasm of these cells. Interestingly, the Golgi region stains relatively stronger than the remainder of the cytoplasm, consistent with the possibility that this is an actively synthesizing cell that secretes the hormone rapidly and retains no storage granules. A few cells, however, retain strong cytoplasmic staining despite hypothyroidism. Eventually, the depleted cells contain one or few large vacuoles with sharply delineated borders, and the reaction to staining for thyrotropic hormone becomes negative except for mild darkening in the Golgi area.

The morphologically similar thyroidectomy and castration cells can be differentiated by staining with peroxidase-labeled antibodies. The positively identified thyroidectomy cells never stain after application of antiluteinizing hormone. Cells that do stain after application of antithyrotropic hormone never develop vacuoles on ovariectomy. The vacuolated castration cells in pituitaries of ovariectomized rats never stain after application of antithyrotropic hormone.

On rebound from thyroid deficiency, the thyroidectomy cell assumes intense staining after application of antithyrotropic hormone.

Thyroidectomy or treatment with propylthiouracil exert profound influence on other pituitary cells. Growth hormone cells are no longer identifiable with antigrowth hormone; prolactin cells are reduced in size and number, but gonadotropin cells continue staining after application of antiluteinizing hormone although the cell size is decreased.

Thyroxin, on the other hand, exerts differential effects on pituitary cells. The thyrotropic hormone cells become unidentifiable immunocytochemically. However, the gonadotropic, prolactin, and corticotropic cells continue to stain after treatment with their specific antihormone sera, although the size of some of these cells may be altered.

The enzyme-labeled antibody method is particularly useful in routine diagnostic tests for autoimmune disease (Chapter 9). Lupus erythematosus is diagnosed by application to cell nuclei (such as obtained in cryostat sections of snap-frozen rat liver) of patient's serum and either fluorescein or peroxidase-conjugated antihuman IgG. Similarly, skin biopsies in pemphigoid lesions have been compared by fluorescein and peroxidase-conjugated antibodies. The granular deposits of immune complex nephritis can be observed in the renal basement membrane by immunofluorescence as well as with peroxidase-conjugated anti-IgG. Autoimmune antibodies can also be demonstrated in ulcerative colitis with peroxidase-conjugated antihuman IgG. In all these applications immunofluorescence and peroxidase-conjugated antibodies are of approximately equal sensitivities. Intrinsic peroxidase activity of tissue may give some nonspecific background in the peroxidase-conjugated antibody method, but Werner Straus has shown that peroxidase can be irreversibly inhibited by methanol containing 1% sodium nitroferricyanate and 1% acetic acid. It is unlikely that this treatment materially affects the reactivity of most tissue antigens. In routine diagnostic procedure, the peroxidase-conjugated antibody method is preferable to immunofluorescence if one wants to avoid the use of a fluorescent microscope and if one wishes to obtain permanent preparations.

Two-Step Conjugation of Peroxidase with Immunoglobulin

As we have seen, many of the problems of cross-linking peroxidase with immunoglobulin by a single-step addition of a bifunctional reagent are due to the difference of rate of reaction of both proteins. The uneven competition of both proteins for reagent can be avoided if the reaction is carried out in two steps: in the first step, peroxidase is reacted with excess of bifunctional reagent so that only one functional group combines, while the other functional group remains unaltered. For the second step uncombined reagent is removed, and the peroxidase conjugated with bifunctional reagent that has one of its functional groups unaltered, is admixed with immunoglobulin to form the peroxidase-immunoglobulin conjugate. This procedure, introduced by S. Avrameas and T. Ternyck, depends on the observation that reaction of peroxidase with an excess of amine-reactive bifunctional reagent does not abolish enzyme activity.

Ten mg of peroxidase are dissolved in 0.2 ml of 0.1 M phosphate buffer, pH 6.8, containing 1.25% glutaraldehyde. The solution is left at room temperature for 18 hours and passed through a Sephadex G-25 column equilibriated with saline. The dark colored eluate fractions are concentrated to 1 ml and added to 1 ml of a 0.5% solution of purified antibody in saline. Following admixture of 0.1 M carbonate buffer, pH 9.5, the solution is left at 4° for 24 hours. After addition of 0.1 ml of a 0.2 M solution of lysine for two hours (to terminate the reaction by inactivation of some of the residual aldehyde), the solution is dialyzed against buffered saline at 4°. The antibody-containing components are separated from any unreacted peroxidase by precipitation with ammonium sulfate. The redissolved, dialyzed material is stored at 4° for one week prior to use.

This procedure resembles the two-stage conjugation of ferritin with immunoglobulin except that in the ferritin method unreacted immunoglobulin is separated from a conjugate mixture still containing unreacted ferritin, while in the present method unreacted peroxidase is separated from a conjugate mixture still containing unreacted immunoglobulin [Fig. 5-6(c)]. Indeed, the bulk of reaction product is unreacted immunoglobulin. If the reaction product is applied to a Sephadex G-200 column, the conjugate proper elutes slightly in front of the unconjugated antibody. Hence, its molecular weight is probably not in excess of 200,000 indicating that, indeed, it consists of one molecule of peroxidase conjugated with a single molecule of antibody and not with a number of molecules of antibody. Thus, the main objective of the two-step conjugation procedure is attained. However, preparative separation of conjugate from unconjugated antibody would entail difficulties, because both charge and weight of the conjugate are fairly close to those of unconjugated immunoglobulin.

When the two-step method is used for conjugation of peroxidase with Fab, conjugate with a molecular weight of 80,000 is obtained consisting of one peroxidase and one Fab molecule. This conjugate is easily separated from unconjugated peroxidase as well as from Fab, which both elute at a molecular weight fraction of 40,000.

Conjugation in two stages can also be done with 2,4-toluene diisocyanate, the bifunctional reagent used in the immunoferritin method (page 59). R. Modesto and A. Pesce have developed an assay for evaluating the amount of reagent bound to protein during conjugation. For cross-linking of peroxidase with immunoglobulin, it is necessary that in the first stage the reagent reacts monofunctionally leaving one isocyanate group free. Bifunctional reaction results in purely intramolecular binding or in polymerization of peroxidase. Free isocyanate can be determined spectrophotometrically after conversion to the amine, diazotization, and azo-coupling. Bound isocyanate can be determined by hydrolysis of the ureido groups, diazotization, and azo-coupling. This analysis has permitted the development of conditions for optimal conjugation of peroxidase with immunoglobulin. Mild conditions are found necessary even for the first reaction step (2,4-diisocyanate with peroxidase) to avoid polymerization of peroxidase. Even under mild conditions some of the reagent is bound intramolecularly in peroxidase, leaving about 0.37 molecules of monofunctionally bound reagent per molecule of peroxidase and affecting enzyme activity only slightly. Despite this mild degree of reaction in the first step, conjugation with immunoglobulin occurs in the second step (admixture of diisocyanate-reacted peroxidase with immunoglobulin). However, polymerization to larger aggregates, so burdensome in single step conjugation procedures, is averted. The peroxidase conjugate contains one molecule of peroxidase reacted with one molecule of immunoglobulin, as its molecular weight is 200,000 by gel filtration. Again, it is difficult to separate the one peroxidase-one immunoglobulin conjugate from unreacted immunoglobulin. The yield of this conjugate is 4%.

Size of Conjugate and Tissue Penetration

The sensitivity of staining is about equal whether two-step or one-step conjugate is used. However, the penetration of formaldehyde-fixed cells is more rapid with two-step-prepared peroxidase-antibody or peroxidase-Fab conjugate than with one-step prepared peroxidase-antibody conjugate. Apparently, the one-step conjugate penetrates slower, because its IgG is polymeric.

The conjugation of peroxidase with Fab in two steps increases penetrability for three reasons:

1. Polymerization of Fab is minimized, and the bulk of conjugate is binary (one peroxidase and one Fab subunit).

2. Substitution of Fab for IgG decreases the size of the binary complex by 120,000 daltons.

3. Conjugated Fab is easily separated from unconjugated Fab.

If tissue penetration is difficult, competition of any unconjugated Fab or IgG for conjugate is exacerbated, because unconjugated material penetrates faster than conjugate (page 86).

To further improve penetrability, cytochrome c (molecular weight 12,500) has been substituted for peroxidase (molecular weight 39,800) by J. P. Kraehenbuhl, P. B. De Grandi, and M. A. Campiche. Horseradish peroxidase at pH 7.0, 37°, possesses an oxidation reduction potential of -0.27 volt. Cytochrome c under the same conditions has an oxidation reduction potential of $+0.26$ volt. Thus, under physiologic conditions cytochrome c is not a peroxidase. Mitochondria usually do not have background staining in immunocytochemical methods that use horseradish peroxidase with diaminobenzidine and hydrogen peroxide. The differences of horseradish peroxidase and cytochrome c suggest that the iron porphyrin is linked to protein in a different manner. T. Flatmark has shown, however, that cytochrome c does exhibit peroxidatic activity below pH 5. Using 1,2,3-trihydroxybenzene as electron donor, the pH optimum is dependent on the nature of the anion present, being highest with citrate (about 3.5). The change in activity with ion concentration follows ordinary dissociation curves, indicating that cytochrome c is dissociably combined with the anions. Furthermore, below pH 5.0 one of the hemochromogen-forming groups becomes ionized, thus, splitting one of the iron protein bonds. Below the pH optimum, apparently, a second iron protein bond is split, and the enzyme is inactivated. At the pH optimum the hematin iron is conceivably heteroligated, forming one bond with the protein and another with the anion. Activity is, therefore, strongly dependent on the nature of the anion. Conceivably, the heteroligated form of cytochrome c at acid pH may resemble horseradish peroxidase at neutral pH. The optimum conditions for peroxidatic activity of cytochrome c are pH 3.5 in 0.12 M citrate buffer. However, even under these conditions about 30 times higher concentrations of hydrogen peroxide (0.3%) are needed to obtain a measurable enzyme reaction than in the case of horseradish peroxidase at neutral pH. The relative velocity of peroxidase to cytochrome c is 6,000 to 0.02 units with o-dianisidine as electron donor. In order to apply diaminobenzidine and hydrogen peroxide to the staining of cytochrome c in tissues, M. J. Karnovsky and D. F. Rice find that at pH 3.9 the concentration of hydrogen peroxide must be reduced to 0.03% to avoid deleterious effects on tissue. One must expect, therefore, that cytochrome c-conjugated antibodies are not as sensitive detectors as horseradish peroxidase-conjugated antibodies.

Diaminobenzidine is rapidly oxidized by hydrogen peroxide at acid pH even in the absence of enzyme. This reaction is, perhaps, trace metal-catalyzed. Citrate buffer as it chelates with the metal may have the added advantage of preventing this spontaneous oxidation.

Kraehenbuhl and co-workers have conjugated cytochrome c with IgG or Fab in a single step glutaraldehyde procedure. Cytochrome c-Fab conjugate was eluted from Sephadex G-100 as the leading, heterogeneous peak with an approximate molecular weight of 70,000. Polymeric and unconjugated cytochrome c were parts of the trailing four peaks. The eluted conjugate (pooled leading peak) probably consisted of one or two Fab units conjugated with one or more cytochrome c units. Cytochrome c seems to be more reactive with glutaraldehyde than horseradish peroxidase. Thus, conjugated and unconjugated polymeric cytochrome c is formed, while in the conjugation procedure for peroxidase polymeric peroxidase is negligible.

There are now available several immunocytochemical reagents of fairly defined size for the study of the effect of size on cell penetrability. They are as follows:

1. Ferritin-conjugated IgG prepared under mild conditions and carefully freed of unconjugated IgG, molecular weight 650,000.

2. Ferritin following application of hybrid antibody, effective molecular weight 500,000.

3. Peroxidase-conjugated IgG, prepared by the single-step glutaraldehyde procedure, consisting of three subunits of IgG and one subunit of peroxidase, molecular weight 500,000.

4. Peroxidase-antiperoxidase complex, molecular weight 400,000 (page 138).

5. Peroxidase-conjugated Fab, prepared by the one-step glutaraldehyde procedure, consisting of two subunits of Fab and one subunit of peroxidase, molecular weight 120,000.

6. Peroxidase-conjugated Fab, prepared by the two-step glutaraldehyde procedure, consisting of one subunit of Fab and one subunit of peroxidase, molecular weight 80,000.

7. Cytochrome c-conjugated Fab, molecular weight approximately 70,000 (the cytochemically effective size of this heterogeneous conjugate may be smaller as it is selectively sieved during penetration of cell membrane barriers).

Peroxidase-conjugated IgG prepared by the one-step FNPS procedure, or the two-step glutaraldehyde, or toluene diisocyanate procedure are not included in the list since the presence of unconjugated immunoglobulin in these preparations may vitiate interpretation of results.

Ingested ferritin can be seen by electron microscopy in vacuoles of the jejunal absorptive cell. J. P. Kraehenbuhl, P. B. De Grandi, and M. A.

Campiche studied the penetration of peroxidase and cytochrome c-conjugated antibody and Fab into the ferritin-containing vacuoles after application to 30–40 μ thick, unfrozen tissue chopper sections and evaluating the enzyme reaction deposits in the vacuoles. Conjugated, purified antiferritin was used in the direct method, conjugated purified anti-IgG or anti-Fab in the indirect method. The degree of penetration was evaluated by estimating the ratio of labeled to unlabeled vacuolar volume. No penetration occurred with any conjugate when the tissue had been fixed in glutaraldehyde. After fixation with paraformaldehyde, a low percentage of labeling was observed in the direct and indirect methods when the molecular weight of the tracers was larger than 200,000. Sixty-eight percent of vacuoles were labeled in the direct method with peroxidase conjugated Fab antiferritin. In the indirect method, which is more sensitive, nearly all vacuoles were labeled with peroxidase or cytochrome c-conjugated sheep Fab antirabbit Fab, provided papain-digested antiferritin preceded the anti-Fab. With peroxidase conjugates some nonspecific deposition of reaction product occurred, especially on nuclei and mitochondria and was more marked with the larger conjugates (see also page 84). Nonspecific localization was not observed when cytochrome c-conjugated Fab was used, but this may conceivably have been due to lesser sensitivity of the cytochrome marker.

It is also worth noting that all hemoproteins do not polymerize diaminobenzidine to the same extent, and that diffusion artifacts from lesser polymerization may occur on acidic structures as observed by Alex Novikoff and his associates. For this reason it is wise to stick to horseradish peroxidase rather than using lesser peroxidases.

REFERENCES

Avrameas, S. Coupling of enzymes to proteins with glutaraldehyde. Use of the conjugates for the detection of antigens and antibodies. *Immunochemistry,* **6**:43, 1969.

Avrameas, S. Immunoenzyme techniques: Enzymes as markers for the localization of antigens and antibodies. *Int. Rev. Cytol.,* **27**:349, 1970.

Avrameas, S. and Guilbert, B. A method for quantitative determination of cellular immunoglobulins by enzyme-labeled antibodies. *Eur. J. Immunol.,* **1**:394, 1971.

Avrameas, S. and Ternyck, T. Peroxidase labeled antibody and FAb conjugates with enhanced intracellular penetration. *Immunochemistry,* **8**:1175, 1971.

Baker, B. L. and Yu, Y. Y. Hypophyseal changes induced by thyroid deficiency and thyroxine administration as revealed by immunochemical staining. *Endocrinology,* 89:996, 1971.

Clyne, D. H., Norris, S. H., Modesto, R. R., Pesce, A. J., and Pollak, V. E. Antibody enzyme conjugates. The preparation of intermolecular conjugates of horseradish peroxidase and antibody and their use in immunohistology of renal cortex. *J. Histochem. Cytochem.,* 21:233, 1973.

De Grandi, P. B., Kraehenbuhl, J. P., and Campiche, M. A. Ultrastructural localization of calcitonin in the parafollicular cells of pig thyroid gland with cytochrome c-labeled antibody fragments. *J. Cell Biol.,* 50:446, 1971.

Dowling, J., Johnson, G. D., Webb, J. A., and Smith, M. E. Use of peroxidase-conjugated antiglobulin as an alternative to immunofluorescence for the detection of antinuclear factor in serum. *J. Clin. Path.,* 24:501, 1971.

Flatmark, T. Studies on the peroxidase effect of cytochrome c. IV. The influence of pH and certain anions on the overall reaction. *Acta Chem. Scand.,* 19:2059, 1965.

Graham, R. C. Jr. and Karnovsky, M. J. The early stages of absorption of injected horseradish peroxidase in the proximal tubules of mouse kidney: ultrastructural cytochemistry by a new technique. *J. Histochem. Cytochem.,* 14:291, 1966.

Hoffman, N. A. and Hartford, P. M. Application of peroxidase-labeled antibodies to the localization of renin. *J. Histochem. Cytochem.,* 19:811, 1971.

Karnovsky, M. J. and Rice, D. F. Exogenous cytochrome c as an ultrastructural tracer. *J. Histochem. Cytochem.,* 17:751, 1969.

Kraehenbuhl, J. P., De Grandi, P. B., and Campiche, M. A. Ultrastructural localization of intracellular antigen using enzyme-labeled antibody conjugates. *J. Cell Biol.,* 50:432, 1971.

Lustig, L., Ultrastructural localization of soluble collagen antigen. *J. Histochem. Cytochem.,* 19:663, 1971.

Machida, M. and Hoshino, M. The ultrastructural localization of antigens in Ehrlich ascitic tumor cells against antinuclear factor in lupus erythematosus sera by peroxidase-labeled antibody method. *Experientia,* 27:201, 1971.

Mednick, M. L., Petrali, J. P., Thomas, N. C., Sternberger, L. A., Plapinger, R. F., Davis, D. A., Wasserkrug, H. L., and Seligman, A M. Localization of acetylcholinesterase via production of osmiophilic polymers: New benzenediazonium salts with thiolacetate functions. *J. Histochem. Cytochem.* 19:155, 1971.

Modesto, R. R. and Pesce, A. J. The reaction of 4,4'-difluoro-3,3'-γ-globulin and horseradish peroxidase. *Biochim. Biophys. Acta,* **229**:384, 1971.

Nakane, P. Application of peroxidase-labeled antibodies to the intracellular localization of hormones. *Acta Endocrinol.* Suppl., **153**:190, 1971.

Nakane, P. K. Classification of anterior pituitary cell types with immunoenzyme histochemistry. *J. Histochem. Cytochem.,* **18**:9, 1970.

Nakane, P. K. Simultaneous localization of multiple tissue antigens using the peroxidase-labeled antibody method: A study on pituitary glands of the rat. *J. Histochem. Cytochem.,* **16**:557, 1968.

Nakane, P. K. and Pierce, G. B., Jr. Enzyme-labeled antibodies for the light and electron microscopic localization of tissue antigens. *J. Cell Biol.,* **33**:307, 1967.

Nakane, P. K. and Pierce, G. B., Jr. Enzyme-labeled antibodies: preparation and application for the localization of antigens. *J. Histochem. Cytochem.,* **14**:929, 1966.

Novikoff, A. B., Novikoff, P. M., Quintana, N., and Davis, C. Diffusion artifacts in 3,3'-diaminobenzidine cytochemistry. *J. Histochem. Cytochem.,* **20**:745, 1972.

Phifer, R. F., Midgley, A. R., and Spicer, S. S. Immunohistologic and histologic evidence that follicle-stimulating hormone and luteinizing hormone are present in the same cell type in the human pars distalis. *J. Clin. Endocrin. Metab.,* **36**:125, 1973.

Seligman, A. M., Karnovsky, M. J., Wasserkrug, H. L., and Hanker, J. S. Nondroplet ultrastructural demonstration of cytochrome oxidase activity with a polymerizing osmiophilic reagent, diaminobenzidine (DAB). *J. Cell Biol.* **38**:1, 1968.

Shnitka, T. K. and Seligman, A. M. Ultrastructural localization of enzymes. *Ann. Rev. Biochem.* **40**:375, 1971.

Straus, W. Inhibition of peroxidase by methanol and by methanol-nitroferricyanate for use in immunoperoxidase procedures. *J. Histochem. Cytochem.,* **19**:682, 1971.

Ubertini, T., Wilkie, B. N., and Noronha, F. Use of horseradish peroxidase-labeled antibody for light and electron microscope localization of reovirus antigen. *Appl. Microbiol.,* **21**:534, 1971.

Chapter 6

The Unlabeled Antibody

Enzyme Method

We have seen in the preceding chapters that problems of specificity of staining with labeled antibodies can usually be attributed to the process of labeling itself. We have also seen that the introduction of an enzymatic label for antibody failed to increase staining sensitivities beyond those of the immunofluorescence and immunoferritin methods, even though an enzyme molecule yields with a histochemical substrate a multitude of visualizable product molecules.

The unlabeled antibody enzyme method seeks to avoid this shortcoming by attaching an enzyme, such as horseradish peroxidase, to tissue antigen via specific antibody without use of a covalent labeling reaction. This has been possible by employing the antibody specific combining property for two different purposes. The first purpose is the same as in the labeled antibody methods; that is, antibody is used directly or indirectly as a reagent for selective localization of the tissue antigen under investigation. However, instead of visualizing this reaction by labeling the antibody, visualization is done by using specific antibody binding a second time, this time to bind onto antibody an enzyme that is detectable by a suitable histochemical substrate. The double use of antibody specificity in sequence depends on the bivalence of IgG.

In the unlabeled antibody enzyme method, as originally used (Fig. 6-1), tissue antigen is localized by application of specific antiserum from species A ("primary antibody"). Since the sensitivity of the method is high, this antiserum can usually be extensively diluted. Under these conditions antibody generally binds via both of its specific combining sites. In the second step antiserum produced in species B against IgG of species A is applied in excess. Because of the excess only one of the combining sites of the anti-IgG attaches, while the second site remains free. In the third step antiperoxidase purified from antiserum produced in species A is applied. The free combining site of the anti-IgG now binds the antiperoxidase. Under

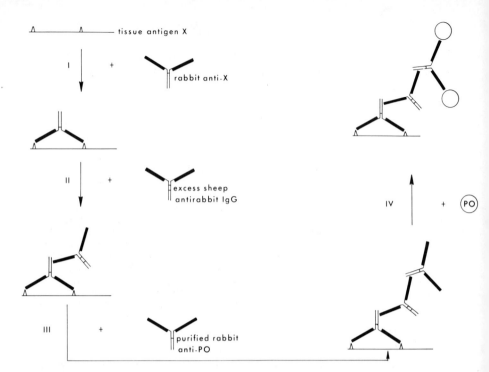

Fig. 6-1 Schematics of the unlabeled antibody enzyme method using purified antiperoxidase. Tissue antigen is localized by the sequential application of antiserum produced in species A (I), antiserum to IgG of species A produced in species B (II), purified antiperoxidase from species A (III), and peroxidase (IV), followed by staining with 4,4'-diaminobenzidine tetrahydrochloride and hydrogen peroxide and by osmication (not shown). The heavy lines in the diagram of the IgG molecule represent its two FAb portions, each containing one L-chain and the N-terminal part of one γ-chain. The two fine lines in each molecule represent the Fc portion consisting of the C-terminal parts of both γ-chains. In rabbit IgG the two γ-chains are bound by a single sulfhydryl linkage. In sheep IgG the γ-chains have been arbitrarily diagrammed as being bound by two sulfhydral linkages. PO, peroxidase. From L. A. Sternberger in *Electron Microscopy of Enzymes: Principles and Methods*, Vol. I, H. M. Hayat (ed.). Von Nostrand Reinhold Co., New York, 1973.

these conditions (where antiperixodase is the antigen) usually both, but in any event at least one of the specific peroxidase combining sites of the antiperoxidase remains free. In the fourth step peroxidase is applied for reaction with the specific combining sites of the bound antiperoxidase. In the fifth step the bound peroxidase is reacted with its substrates, hydrogen peroxide, and diaminobenzidine. Enzyme action forms the insoluble, polymeric oxidation product of diaminobenzidine that is brown in light microscopy and invisible in electron microscopy. In the sixth step this product reacts with osmium tetroxide to form an insoluble, amorphous chelate that is black in light microscopy and opaque in electron miscroscopy.

Purified antiperoxidase is needed, because IgG of specificities other than antiperoxidase blocks reaction of antiperoxidase in the fourth step. Unfortunately, the preparation of antiperoxidase by specific immunoabsorbents is less efficient a procedure than that of most other antiprotein antibodies. The reason is an unusually low dissociability of the peroxidase-antiperoxidase bond, even at acid pH (Fig. 6-2). If treatment at pH 2.3 is carried out at 1°, practically no antibody is recovered. Yield improves with rise in temperature and increase in time of acid treatment with incumbent danger of denaturation of antibody. Upon brief dissociation at room temperature, denaturation is insignificant, but only a fraction of the total antibody is eluted from the immunoabsorbent. Unfortunately, this fraction con-

Fig. 6-2 Solubilization by acid dissociation of antiperoxidase from a peroxidase-antiperoxidase precipitate or peroxidase immunoabsorbent. At pH 2.3 the equilibrium of bound and free antiperoxidase tends towards the bound state (upper part of figure). Yield of free antiperoxidase (purified antibody) increases with increase in temperature and dilution. In general only that fraction of antibody is obtained in solution that possesses the poorest avidity for peroxidase. If, however, free peroxidase is added to the acid dissociation mixture, the free antiperoxidase is bound with peroxidase in solution-forming peroxidase-antiperoxidase complex (PAP) solubilized by excess peroxidase (lower part of figure). Just as the equilibrium of reaction favors the immune precipitate or absorbent-bound form of antiperoxidase at pH 2.3, so does it favor its binding with added peroxidase as soluble peroxidase-antiperoxidase complex. The formation of peroxidase-antiperoxidase complex removes the free form of antiperoxidase from the solubilization reaction equilibrium, so that more free peroxidase can dissociate from the precipitate or immunoabsorbent. The yield-limiting factor in this reaction is the degree of excess of added peroxidase. However, even a small amount of free peroxidase yields some soluble peroxidase-antiperoxidase complex, since even a small amount is excess to the very small amount of antiperoxidase that is free in solution at any time. Since the binding of antiperoxidase with free peroxidase is "equi-avid" to that in the immune precipitate or absorbent, the proportion of high and low avidity antiperoxidase in PAP is the same as that of the original peroxidase-antiperoxidase precipitate or absorbent. From the work of L. A. Sternberger.

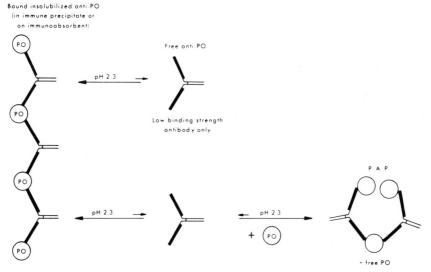

Bound insolubilized anti-PO
(in immune precipitate or
on immunoabsorbent)

PO

Free anti PO

pH 2 3

Low binding strength
antibody only

PO

PO

P A P

pH 2 3

pH 2 3

PO

+ free PO

High and low binding strength
antibody obtained

sists of the antibodies with the weakest avidities (pages 2 and 15) for peroxidase, leaving those species of antibodies with stronger avidities on the immunoabsorbent. In immunocytochemistry usually an excess of antibody is applied to antigen in the specimen. This assures that antibodies with the strongest avidities are bound preferentially, while the weaker antibodies stay in solution. Dissociation during washing is thereby minimized. In step three of the unlabeled antibody enzyme method, however, antiperoxidase is applied as antigen to anti-IgG bound in the specimen. The tightness of this bond is a reflection of the avidity of the anti-IgG for IgG and not of the antiperoxidase for peroxidase. Hence, there can be no selection for antiperoxidase with high avidity. Indeed, when purified antiperoxidase is used, the binding strength of the antibody is so poor that much of the peroxidase reacted in step four is lost in the subsequent steps along with the enzyme reaction product (dissociation during immunohistochemical staining is further discussed on pages 176 and 182). Also, a relatively large amount of peroxidase is needed for preparation of immunoabsorbents to yield a relatively small amount of purified antibody.

To obviate the low yields and especially the low avidities of antibodies eluted from immunoabsorbents, a moderate excess of peroxidase can be added to immune precipitates during dissociation at pH 2.3. In the absence of added peroxidase, the concentration of free antibody and free peroxidase dissociated from precipitates is low even at acid pH. Any fraction of precipitate that has dissociated tends to recombine and reincorporate into the precipitate. Addition of a moderate excess of free peroxidase, however, is sufficient to prevent precipitation upon recombination of free antibody with peroxidase, since antigen-antibody complexes containing an excess of antigen are soluble (page 9). As the avidity of the dissociated antibody is equal for a molecule of peroxidase in the precipitate and in solution, the added peroxidase competes effectively with the precipitate for free antibody. Thus in the presence of a sufficient excess of peroxidase, an immune precipitate will dissolve instantaneously at pH 2.3 at 1°. When a small excess of peroxidase is added, solution of the precipitate is partial. The product of acid dissociation with added peroxidase is, of course, purified, soluble peroxidase-antiperoxidase complex (PAP) rather than purified antiperoxidase. Importantly, no selection is made in the preparation of PAP against antibodies with high avidity. Indeed, PAP posses higher overall binding avidity for antigen than most other antigen-antibody complexes (page 140).

In the staining sequence by the unlabeled antibody enzyme method, PAP possesses a dual function: it has enzymatic activity and is an antigen reactive with the anti-IgG attached to the tissue site (Fig. 6-3). It is important that peroxidase activity is not abolished in PAP. In general, antibodies reacting with enzymes impair though rarely abolish enzymatic activity, even if reaction occurs in antibody excess. In PAP impairment of peroxidase activity varies from 2–30%. Peroxidase activity is not affected by the acid conditions used for the preparation of PAP. Neither is peroxidase activity hindered sterically, although activity *is* affected in peroxidase-antiperoxidase complexes of lower antigen-antibody ratios. Most probably the observed loss of activity in PAP is due to sodium ions during storage. Since this loss is small, it is inconsequential for immunocytochemical measurements.

Fig. 6-3 The use of peroxidase-antiperoxidase complex (PAP) simplifies the staining sequence of the unlabeled antibody enzyme method and assures that the peroxidase is firmly bound to the specific tissue sites *via* the intervening antibody reagents. Step I: diluted antiserum from species A specific to tissue constituent X. Step II: excess of antiserum to IgG of species A, produced in species B. Step III: PAP. Steps IV and V (not shown): diaminobenzidine tetrahydrochloride—hydrogen peroxide and osmium tetroxide. From the work of L. A. Sternberger.

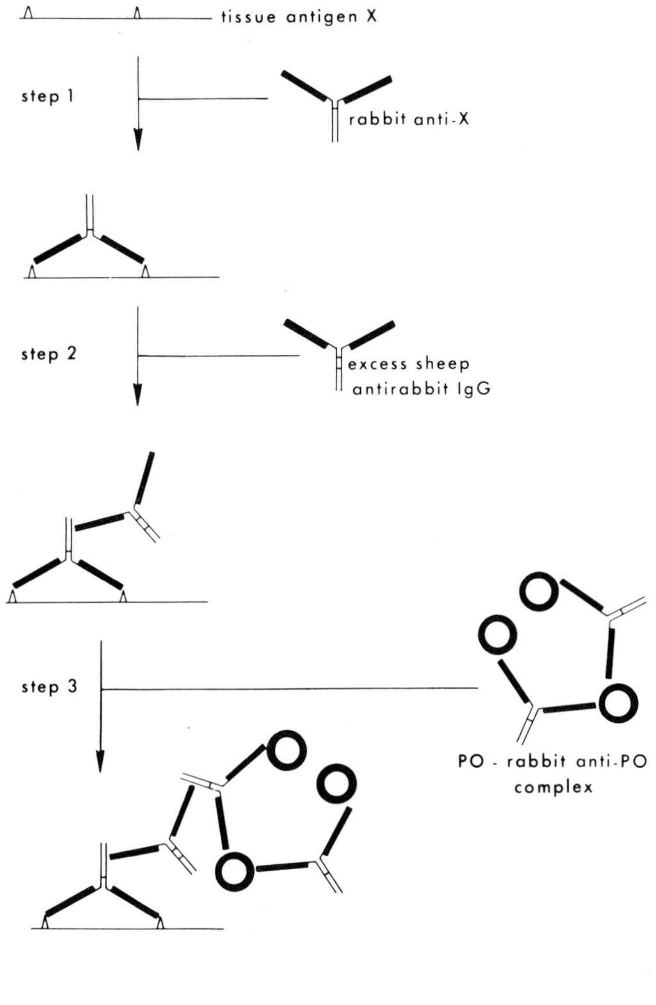

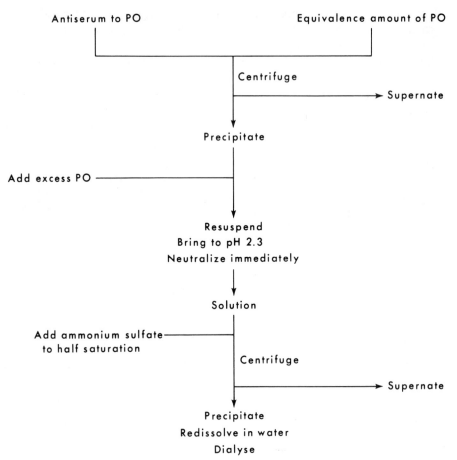

Fig. 6-4 Preparation of immunospecifically purified soluble peroxidase-antiperoxidase complex. From L. A. Sternberger, P. H. Hardy, Jr., J. J. Cuculis, and H. G. Meyer, *J Histochem. Cytochem.*, **18:**315, 1970.

Preparation of PAP is an economical procedure both in peroxidase and in antiperoxidase. Immune precipitates are obtained from antiserum by addition of peroxidase (Fig. 6-4). The washed precipitates are resuspended in saline containing four times the amount of peroxidase used for precipitation, and the suspension is brought to pH 2.3. Following fairly immediate neutralization and removal of any undissociated precipitate, the soluble peroxidase-antiperoxidase complex is separated from free peroxidase by precipitation with ammonium sulfate.

When the original precipitation of antiperoxidase from antiserum is carried out with an amount of peroxidase that precipitates at the antigen excess end of the equivalence zone (amount of peroxidase that precipitates all precipitating antibody from the antiserum and leaves a barely detectable amount of free peroxidase in solution), then the yield of PAP will be about 30% in antibody and 30% in peroxidase. The average molecular ratio of peroxidase to antiperoxidase in PAP will be 3:2. If the original precipitation is done further in antibody excess (and again four times the added amount of peroxidase is used for resuspension), the yield of PAP will be lower in antibody and higher in peroxidase (approximating 100% in peroxidase). The average composition still will be 3:2. If the original precipitation is done further in antigen excess, the yield will be higher in antiperoxidase (approximating 100%) and lower in peroxidase. In this case the immune precipitate will always dissolve completely and instantaneously at pH 2.3. The average composition of PAP will still be 3:2.

The materials lost in preparation of PAP are peroxidase-antiperoxidase precipitate and free peroxidase. Both could be recycled. The material lost in the preparation of antiperoxidase is immunoabsorbent to which the high avidity antibody is still attached. The immunoabsorbent becomes a reagent of lesser and lesser efficiency upon recycling with fresh serum.

The relatively low variance of composition of PAP, the possibility of obtaining it with relatively low excesses of antigen, and a number of other properties discussed on page 136 are the result of unusually stable antigen-antibody bonds. The stability of the complex is a fortunate property that has contributed to the sensitivity of the unlabeled antibody enzyme method and has eventually facilitated its quantitation (Chapter 7).

Preparation of Soluble Peroxidase-Antiperoxidase Complex (PAP): Procedure

In a preliminary test determine qualitatively the equivalence zone of the antiperoxidase serum used [prepared by immunization of rabbits with peroxidase (RZ = 3.0) and Freund's adjuvants]. Place into a series of 10 tubes 0.2 ml saline containing amounts of peroxidase varying from 0.05 to 0.5 mg/ml. Add to each tube 0.2 ml of antiperoxidase serum. Leave tubes at 1–5° C overnight. Centrifuge. Collect supernates into a second set of tubes and transfer 0.15 ml of each supernate from the second set into a third set of tubes. Add to each tube of the second set 0.1 ml of the antiperoxidase serum and observe excess of antigen by qualitatively reading precipitation after one hour at room temperature. Add to each tube of the third set 0.1 ml of a solution of peroxidase (0.1 mg/ml) and observe excess of antibody by qualitatively reading precipitation after one hour. Three zones will be observed: supernates in the zone of excess antibody, supernates in the equivalence zone that show neither excess antibody nor excess antigen, and supernates in the excess antigen zone. Record the concentration of peroxidase *per ml* used in that tube of the equivalence zone that is nearest to the antigen excess zone (AgX equivalence proportion).

Good yields of PAP (in peroxidase as well as in antiperoxidase) are obtained if antiperoxidase is precipitated from antiserum with about 1.5 times AgX equivalence proportion. It is convenient to use 12 mg of peroxidase for this initial precipitation. We now have to determine how much antiserum to use. If 12 mg is 1.5 times AgX equivalence proportion, then 8 mg is AgX equivalence proportion. Assume that in the preliminary test AgX equivalence proportion was recorded in the tube in which 0.4 mg peroxidase per ml (0.08 mg per tube) had been added to antiserum. Then a total of 20 ml antiperoxidase will be needed to precipitate 8 mg peroxidase at the AgX equivalence proportion or 12 mg at 1.5 times AgX equivalence proportion.

Therefore, place in a 250 ml centrifuge bottle 6.0 ml of a 1:500 solution of peroxidase freshly prepared by dissolving 64 mg of lyophylized peroxidase (RZ = 3.0) in 32 ml of saline. Add 20 ml antiperoxidase serum. Mix. Allow to stand at room temperature for one hour. Centrifuge at about 2,000 rpm (International rotor 259) for 20 minutes at 1-5° C. Remove supernate by suction. Resuspend precipitate in a small volume of cold saline by forcing it several times through a 10 ml pipette. Then wash by adding approximately 150 ml of saline. Centrifuge. Carry out a total of three such washes. Thoroughly resuspend precipitate (by forcing it through a pipette) in 24 ml of the 1:500 solution of peroxidase. Under mild stirring bring to pH 2.3 at room temperature with 1.0, 0.1, and 0.01 N hydrochloric acid (1 drop of 1.0 N hydrochloric acid followed by sufficient amounts of the more dilute solutions for fine adjustment). Neutralize fairly immediately to approximately pH 7.4, using sodium hydroxide solutions (1.0, 0.1, and 0.01 N). Add 2.4 ml of a solution containing 0.08 N sodium acetate and 0.15 N ammonium acetate. Chill solution on an ice bath. Centrifuge at approximately 17,500 rpm for eight minutes at 1° C (Sorvall rotor SS-34). Carry out all subsequent steps in refrigerated containers at 0–2° C or in a cold room at 0–5° C. Under stirring add slowly to the supernate an equal volume of a solution of ammonium sulfate saturated at 0–5° C. Keep stirring for 25 minutes. Centrifuge at 17,500 rpm for 16 minutes at 1° C. Wash precipitate once in half saturated ammonium sulfate solution. Dissolve precipitate in 24 ml of water and dialyze under protection from light against three changes of 15 liter each of sodium ammonium acetate saline (13.5 liter saline, 1.5 liter water, 75 ml of 1.5 N sodium acetate, and 75 ml of 3 N ammonium acetate solution). Centrifuge at 17,500 rpm for 16 minutes. Place 0.1 ml or smaller portions of the supernate into tightly stoppered glass vials held on an ice bath. Freeze in dry ice and acetone and store at or below $-20°$ C in the dark. The peroxidase and anti-peroxidase contents of PAP are determined by absorbence at 400 and 280 m μ of samples diluted 1:5.

Peroxidase (PO) contents of PAP per ml $= OD_{400} \cdot 0.413 \cdot 5$ mg

Anti-PO contents of PAP per ml $=$

$$\left[(OD_{280} \text{ of PAP}) - \frac{(OD_{400} \text{ of PAP}) \cdot (OD_{280} \text{ of PO})}{(OD_{400} \text{ of PO})} \right] \cdot 0.620 \cdot 5 \text{ mg}$$

$$\text{PO/anti-PO mole ratio} = \frac{\text{mg PO} \cdot 156,000}{\text{mg anti-PO} \cdot 39,800}$$

PAP is prepared from antiperoxidase serum of the animal species that donates the antiserum reacting with the localized tissue antigen. Dougherty, Marucci, and DiStefano find that special conditions have to be followed in the preparation of PAP from chicken antisera. Admixture of an equivalent amount of peroxidase rapidly forms a precipitate which, because of its gelatinous nature, has to be resuspended after each centrifugation by treatment for 5 to 15 seconds with a needle probe oscillator, such as "Biosonic II." During dialysis of redissolved chicken PAP, after the ammonium sulfate precipitation step a voluminous, white precipitate forms. This precipitate, which is discarded, contains only a trace of peroxidase and only a small fraction of total globulin. Apparently, the precipitate is related to a non-specific protein known to coprecipitate with avian immune precipitates.

Properties of Soluble
Peroxidase-Antiperoxidase Complex (PAP)

Conventionally, soluble antigen-antibody complexes are prepared by shaking washed precipitates with excess antigen for prolonged periods at neutral pH. Large excesses of antigen are needed, and considerable denaturation occurs. Alternatively, soluble complexes can be prepared by adding excess antigen to purified antibody, if available. PAP, on the other hand, is prepared by near instantaneous exchange of a moderate excess of antigen with immune precipitates at acid pH.

Conventionally-prepared bovine serum albumin - antibovine serum albumin complexes consist of heterogeneous mixtures of complexes of two antigen molecules and one antibody molecule (Ag_2Ab), three antigen and two antibody molecules (Ag_3Ab_2) and, presumably, linear complexes of larger sizes, such as Ag_4Ab_3, Ag_5Ab_4 that are difficult to separate from each other. Large excess of free antigen is needed to maintain these complexes. Upon separation from free antigen, such as occurs in zonal centrifugation,

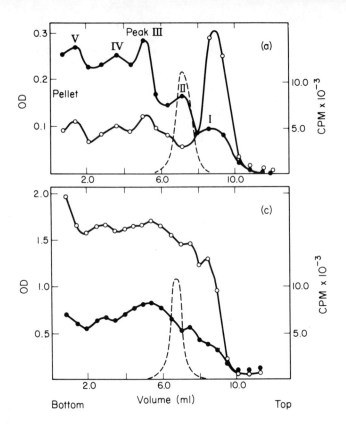

the complexes dissociate rapidly, and free antibody, $AgAb_1$, and $AgAb_2$ become the major components. Apparently, only a high concentration of free antigen assures presence of appreciable amounts of Ag_3Ab_2 and, especially, Ag_2Ab.

On the other hand, PAP with an average composition of peroxidase to antiperoxidase of 3:2 gives an ultracentrifugation a major peak at 11.5 S using Schlieren optics. The peak corresponds to a molecular weight of 400,000 to 429,000 or complexes consisting of three peroxidase and two antiperoxidase molecules. It must be assumed that free antigen is also present since equilibria exist between antigen-antibody complexes of varying composition in solution and since free antigen is needed to maintain the complexes in solution and prevent formation of complexes of lower antigen-antibody ratios that would precipitate. The necessary concentration of free antigen is often too small to be detected by the relatively insensitive Schlieren optics.

In boundary sedimentation a solution of uniform composition is placed into the ultracentrifuge cell, and its constituents are allowed to sediment away from the meniscus. Peroxidase-antiperoxidase complex sediments faster than free peroxidase. As a consequence, any free peroxidase necessary to maintain PAP in solution is in the solvent surrounding the boundary of sedimenting PAP throughout the course of ultracentrifugation. On the

138

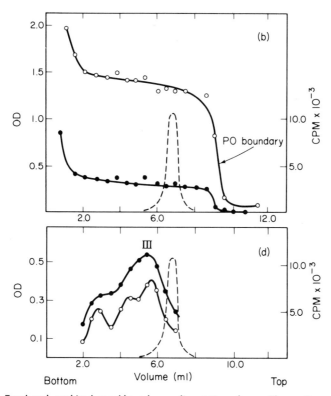

Fig. 6-5 Zonal and combined zonal-boundary sedimentation of peroxidase-antiperoxidase complex (PAP) on continuous sucrose density gradients. Peroxidase concentration was measured by absorbence (OD) at 404 nm (O), protein concentration (immunoglobulin plus peroxidase) by absorbence at 280 nm (●). Broken lines represent position of an ^{125}I-IgG marker. CPM, ^{125}I counts per minute X 10^{-3}. When PAP is applied to the top of a zonal gradient (a), the heavier complex separates upon sedimentation from the lighter free peroxidase that remains close to the top of the gradient (peak I). Lacking any free peroxidase to maintain its composition, the sedimenting PAP reequilibrates forming heavier components. Nevertheless, the 3:2 (peroxidase/antiperoxidase) complex is still the major component with a sedimentation coefficient of 11 (peak III). However, heavier peaks (IV and V) and a 2:1 peak (II) are also prominent. In addition some of the complex precipitates as a pellet. In order to maintain free peroxidase throughout sedimentation, a concentration of 0.58 mg peroxidase per ml was admixed to the gradient-establishing sucrose. On sedimentation of this mixture alone (b), a boundary becomes established below which the concentration of peroxidase remains fairly constant. On addition of PAP to the top of such a gradient (c), the sedimentation pattern becomes zonal with regard to PAP and remains boundary with regard to peroxidase. Subtraction of the absorbencies in (b) from those in (c) yields the absorbence of PAP in the presence of free peroxidase (d). Now most of the complex is in a single peak that sediments at 11 S. Only part of the complex forms a heavier component, but there is no material corresponding to peak V in (a) and there is no pellet. From the work of D. M. Hinton, W. G. Kavanagh, and L. A. Sternberger.

other hand in zonal sedimentation, as attained by placing PAP as a band on top of a sucrose gradient, the heavier PAP and the lighter peroxidase sediment as separate bands. Therefore, if free peroxidase is necessary to keep PAP in solution, the separation of PAP from peroxidase during sedimentation entails reequilibration of PAP to reform the required free peroxidase. Indeed on zonal sedimentation, reequilibration does occur. Although the complex consisting of three peroxidase and two antiperoxidase molecules is still the major single component even in the absence of free peroxidase, there are two heavier peaks and, in addition, a pellet of insoluble precipitate separates [Fig. 6-5(a)].

On the other hand, if peroxidase is admixed with the sucrose that forms the gradient and PAP is placed on top of the gradient, then sedimentation is still zonal with regard to PAP but is boundary with regard to free peroxidase. The boundary of peroxidase that establishes itself is determined in a control gradient devoid of PAP [Fig. 6-5 (b)]. The PAP, as it sediments as a zone into such a gradient, is surrounded by a known amount of free peroxidase at any location in the sedimentation tube [Fig. 6-5 (c)]. Subtraction of the concentration of free peroxidase from the total concentration at any point in the sedimentation tube gives the concentration of peroxidase-antiperoxidase complex at that point [Fig. 6-5 (d)]. Now most of the peroxidase-antiperoxidase complex retains its sedimentation velocity at approximately 11 S. There is some contamination with a heavier component but, importantly, there is no pellet, indicating that the free peroxidase maintains the complex in solution.

The amount of free peroxidase necessary to maintain PAP in solution may vary with antibodies from different sera. At times it has been immeasurably small. Thus, 99.9% of enzymatic activity in PAP prepared from rabbit serum has been precipitated by sheep serum antirabbit IgG. On other occasions, however, reequilibriation of ammonium sulfate-precipitated PAP after dialysis has been indicated by incomplete reprecipitation in half-saturated ammonium sulfate of the absorbence at 404 nm (absorption maximum for peroxidase).

The fact that PAP, in contrast to other soluble antigen-antibody complexes, can be maintained in solution with small amounts of free peroxidase indicates strong binding of peroxidase and antiperoxidase. Repeat precipitation of PAP (prepared with radioiodinated peroxidase) in half-saturated ammonium sulfate solution and measurement of free and bound peroxidase established the association constant of PAP as 10^8. The unusual stability of PAP is important in its cytochemical use.

On negative staining the predominant form of PAP is ring shaped. Pentagons with diameters of 21 nm are characteristic (Fig. 6-6). Some forms are quadrangular or hexagonal. Occasional linear forms are also seen. When complexes appear as large aggregates on the electron microscopy grid, they seem again to consist of circular subunits of the pentagonal and quadrangular forms. The large aggregates are probably an artifact of drying on the grid. The preponderance of circular forms indicates that ring closure must have given the complex unusual stability. Hexagonal forms may contain four and quadrangular forms two peroxidase molecules and two antibody molecules. These forms would have molecular weights similar to that

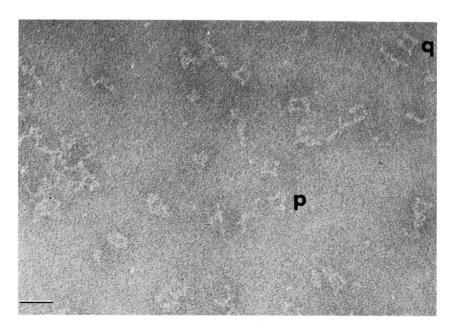

Fig. 6-6 On negative staining of peroxidase-antiperoxidase complex (PAP) ring forms predominate. These rings are usually pentagonal (p), occasionally quadrangular (q) and rarely hexagonal. The diameter of these rings is about 21 nm. Ring closure gives PAP a stability in excess of that of soluble complexes of other antigens and their specific antibodies. The larger aggregates seem to be mainly composed of unit size circular monomers, suggesting that they are due to mechanical aggregation of the circular units upon drying on the grid and not due to antigen-antibody bonding. Marker, 30 nm. This micrograph was taken by Dr. Dennis Brown.

of the 3:2 complex and could have escaped detection by the methods of analysis used.

When soluble complexes are prepared in a manner similar to PAP except for substitution of apoperoxidase for peroxidase (apoperoxidase is peroxidase devoid of heme), a larger excess of apoperoxidase is needed to keep the complex in solution. The conformation of apoperoxidase-antiperoxidase complex differs from that of PAP (Fig. 6-7). There are many small molecules (diameter 3 nm) representing the excess of apoperoxidase needed to keep the complex in solution. In addition there are units of 12 nm diameter with solid cores. Although these units possess the approximate size of IgG, they do not exhibit the typical trilobal conformation of free IgG. Conceivably, these units represent complexes of one or two apoperoxidase and one antiperoxidase molecules. There are no circular forms that would contribute to stability. Perhaps, any larger aggregates if formed have precipitated from solution. Indeed, preparation of apoperoxidase-antiperoxidase complex is a low-yield procedure, requiring very high excesses of apoperoxidase. Apparently, the factors that contribute to the unusual stability of PAP are absent.

141

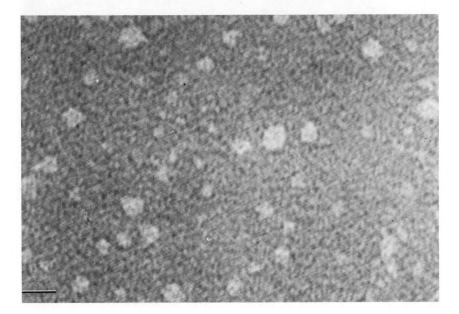

Fig. 6-7 When antigen antibody complex is made by acid dissociation of apoperoxidase-antiperoxidase precipitates in excess of apoperoxidase, a larger excess of antigen is needed to keep the complex soluble than in the case of PAP. The small units (3 nm diameter) are free apoperoxidase molecules. The larger units (12 nm diameter) approximate the dimensions of single antibody molecules. Apparently, they are complexes of one or two apoperoxidase molecules with one antiperoxidase molecule. The apoperoxidase may have masked some of the subunit structure of IgG. Marker, 15 nm. This micrograph was taken by Dr. Dennis Brown.

The tendency to form ring-shaped complex, which apparently is unique to the peroxidase-antiperoxidase system, may conceivably be due to a relatively small number of antigenic determinants in a peroxidase molecule and the placement of these determinants in such a relative position to each other that minimal strain on the angle in the hinge region of IgG occurs when the peroxidase binds to antibody with ring closure. Complexes of 3:2 and 4:2 composition contain, besides peroxidase-antibody bonds, also peroxidase-peroxidase bonds [Fig. 6-8 (a) and (b)].

Peroxidase has been shown to dimerize on acid treatment. This cannot be, however, the cause of ring closure in PAP since the dimerization is fairly rapidly reversed on neutralization. Yet it is possible that even at neutral pH an equilibrium exists between monomeric and a small amount of dimeric forms of peroxidase, and that the spacial conformation of two IgG molecules shifts the equilibrium towards the dimeric form by promoting formation of ring-shaped complexes that contain dimeric peroxidase.

A complex consisting of an equal number of molecules of peroxidase and antiperoxidase is expected to precipitate on linear polymerization.

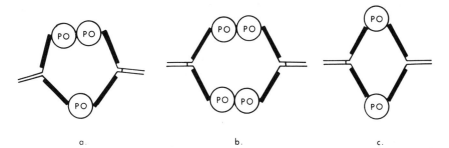

Fig. 6-8 The average peroxidase-antiperoxidase complex consists of three peroxidase (PO) and two anti-PO molecules. The sedimentation velocity of the major component of the complex as well as the size on electron microscopy suggests the conformation A in which two of the PO molecules are dimerized. However admixture with 4 PO — 2 anti-PO complexes (b), 2 PO — 2 anti-PO complexes, (c) and some free PO not necessarily alter the measured average composition. The molecular weights of (b) and (c) are not detectably different from that of (a), nor are the measured dimensions of the rings. Complex (b) in which all the PO molecules are dimerized and (c) in which they are singlets could have hexagonal, respectively quadrangular shapes. From the work of Dennis Hinton, Dennis Brown, and Ludwig Sternberger.

However, a circular complex consisting of only two molecules of peroxidase and two molecules of antiperoxidase [Fig. 6-8(c)] cannot polymerize and remains in solution. Such a complex is suggested by the quadrangular form of PAP in Fig. 6-6.

STAINING FOR LIGHT MICROSCOPY AND PREEMBEDDING STAINING FOR ELECTRON MICROSCOPY

Preparation of cells or tissues is analogous to that of other immunocytochemical methods. For step I (Fig. 6-3) diluted sera can usually be employed. Rabbit, goat, hamster, and chicken sera have been used. For step II sheep or goat serum antirabbit IgG, or rabbit serum antigoat, antihamster, or antichicken IgG have been used respectively. They were employed undiluted or at dilutions up to 1:100. The sera of step II must be used in excess, so that one of the specific combining sites of each reacted antibody remains free. Hence, diluted sera should be used only if their high potency is assured. For step III the PAP is prepared from rabbit or goat serum antiperoxidase or, as in the work of R. Dougherty, A. Marucci, and H. DiStefano, from hamster or chicken serum antiperoxidase, respectively. PAP usually contains 1 to 6 mg antiperoxidase and 0.4 to 2.4 mg peroxidase per ml. PAP has been used undiluted or diluted up to 1:500. Following quick thawing of PAP (water bath at 37°), dilutions are made shortly before use. Diluted PAP is not reused.

As diluents for the reagents in steps I, II, and III, neutral isotonic buffer containing 0.1% gelatin is used or, following the recommendation of L. H. Pratt and R. A. Coleman, normal serum from the same species as the antiserum used in step II.

Incubation times ranging from 10–30 minutes have been used. Shorter incubation times are conceivably possible for surface antigens and longer incubation times as well as correspondingly prolonged wash cycles are needed for preembedding staining of intracellular antigens for electron microscopy. Any neutral buffer or even unbuffered saline are suitable for washing. However, 0.05 M Tris buffer, pH 7.6, must be used for the last wash after step III.

In step IV a freshly prepared solution of 0.05% 3,3'-diaminobenzidine tetrahydrochloride and 0.01% hydrogen peroxide in 0.05 M Tris buffer, pH 7.6, is used for five minutes followed by washing in water or saline (if the pH is more acidic the solution turns brown spontaneously, and staining may be poor). If the staining is too intense, higher dilutions of diaminobenzidine tetrahydrochloride and hydrogen peroxide may be attempted.

For step V, 1% buffered osmium tetroxide is used.

SENSITIVITY

Unstained *Treponema pallidum* is invisible in bright field microscopy as the width of the spirochete is below the resolution of the light microscope. The organism becomes strongly stained in light microscopy upon application of dilutions of rabbit antisyphilitic serum and the unlabeled antibody enzyme method. The titers of several antisera were compared with indirect immunofluorescence (page 38, Table 2-1) and found to be 100–1,000 times higher in the unlabeled antibody enzyme method.

Fig. 6-9 (Opposite page.) Lysozyme in chick embryo cartilage localized by immunofluorescence (a) and by light microscopy with the unlabeled antibody enzyme method (b). Staining occurred in a rim about the chondrocytes in both methods, but higher sensitivity of the unlabeled antibody enzyme method is indicated by additional, less intense, diffuse staining of the intervening cartilage matrix. The perichondrium (upper part of b) does not stain. X500. From K. E. Kuettner, R. Eisenstein, L. W. Soble, and C. Arsenis, *J. Cell Biol.*, **49**:410, 1971. (c) An araldite-embedded Paneth cell stained for lysozyme on the section by the unlabeled antibody enzyme method. Antilysozyme was diluted 1:1,000 and the PAP, originally containing 3.33 mg antiperoxidase and 1.25 mg peroxidase, was diluted 1:50. Lysozyme is revealed in the granules, some of which are in the process of exocytosis (arrows), in the Golgi region (G), in some of the lysozymes (L), and on the microvillar brush border. The brush border of adjacent cells (not shown) also reveals lysozyme. During exocytosis the granules, apparently, fuse with the cell membrane and spill their contents into the intestinal lumen. Residual lysozyme in exocytosing granules is seen as an electron-opaque core within granules possessing an electron-lucid periphery. Lysozymes are pleomorphic structures that, depending on the stage of secretory activity, may or may not contain lysozyme. X5400. From the work of Stanley Erlandsen and Jonathan Parsons.

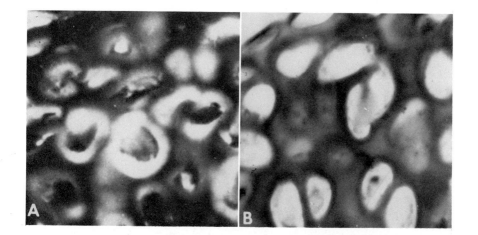

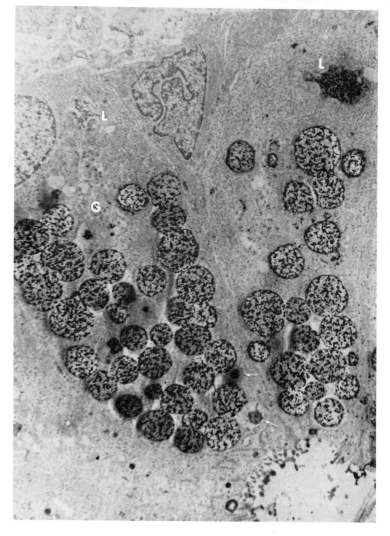

Gwen Moriarty and N. S. Halmi stained on the ultrathin section anterior pituitary corticotropin cells from the same tissue block with various dilutions of anticorticotropin (anti-$\beta_p{}^{17-39}$ ACTH) followed by the enzyme-conjugated and the unlabeled antibody enzyme methods. Electron microscopic localization of the secretion granules by the enzyme-conjugated method had become questionable when the antiserum dilution was 1:100. Most granules remained unstained, and others were weakly stained. On the other hand, the unlabeled antibody enzyme method still gave good localization at an antiserum dilution of 1:500 (anticorticotropin had been applied for two to three minutes).

Gwen Moriarty and her associates also found that the titer of anticorticotropin by unlabeled antibody enzyme electron microscopy is 1,000 times higher than by radioimmunoassay (page 183).

Kuettner, Eisenstein, Soble, and Arsenis demonstrated by immunofluorescence and by the unlabeled antibody enzyme method that chick embryo cartilage lysozyme is primarily extracellular in location (Fig. 6-9a and b). With immunofluorescence, specific localization was intense in a rim about the chondrocytes corresponding to the anatomic lacunae. With the unlabeled antibody enzyme method, the strongest staining occurred in the same location, but increased sensitivity was demonstrated by additional staining though of lesser intensity in the intervening cartilage matrix. Electron microscopy revealed the staining as mainly in the lacunae, surrounding the chondrocytes. The collagen fiber-containing cartilage matrix contained lysozyme only near the lacunar space, and the chondrocyte proper was free of lysozyme.

As in the case of many cancer viruses, tumor and virus-specific antigens can also be differentiated in the avian leukosis group (ALV). *Type specific* (*ts*) antigens induce virus-neutralizing antibodies that react with the viral envelope and are specific to the serotype of the virus used for immunization. Antibodies to *group specific* (*gs*) antigens develop in hamsters bearing tumors induced by the virus. The specificity of these antibodies seems to be independent of the serotype of the virus that has induced the tumor. Tolerance (page 208) to *ts* and *gs* antigens develops in congenitally infected chickens. If these chickens are injected with virus of a different serotype several weeks after hatching, *ts* antibodies specific for this second serotype develop but no *gs* antibodies. Hamster sera containing *gs* antibodies but no *ts* antibodies and chicken sera containing *ts* but no *gs* antibodies are, thus, available.

ALV sometimes exists as a latent virus in otherwise normal chicken cells. Group-specific antigen is an expression of the latent viral genome and is inherited as a genetic factor in inbred lines of chickens.

It has been widely held that animals, in general, are tolerant to *gs* antigens that express a latent cancer virus. This assumption is partly based on the failure to detect *gs* antibodies in immunized chickens by immunofluo-

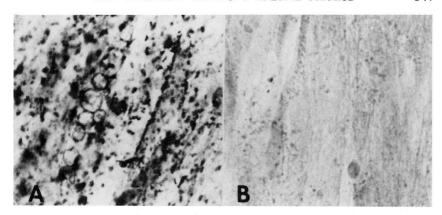

Fig. 6-10 Chick embryo fibroblasts infected with A, a type A strain and B, a type B strain avian leukosis virus, fixed and defatted prior to treatment with strictly type specific chicken serum antitype A (diluted 1:10), rabbit serum antichicken immunoglobulin, chicken PAP and staining for peroxidase. Viral antigen in the interior as well as the exterior of the type A infected cell is stained, while the type specific antigen in the type B infected cell remains unstained. Intracellular reaction product is in the cytoplasm as granules or around vesicles. From the work of R. M. Dougherty, A. A. Marucci, and H. S. DiStefano, *J. Gen. Virol.*, **15**:149, 1972.

Fig. 6-11 Living chick embryo fibroblasts infected with A, a type A strain and B, a type B strain avian leukosis virus and treated with strictly type specific chicken serum antitype B (diluted 1:10). The cells were then fixed and defatted and treated with rabbit serum antichicken immunoglobulin and chicken PAP and stained for peroxidase. The cells infected with type-heterologous virus remain unstained (A). Only the viral antigen on the surface of the type-homologous virus-infected cell accepts the stain, since antibody does not penetrate the cell membrane of living cells. The reaction product appears as long, regular, unbroken coverings on the cell surface. From R. M. Dougherty, A. A. Marucci, and H. S. DiStefano, *J. Gen. Virol.*, **15**:149, 1972.

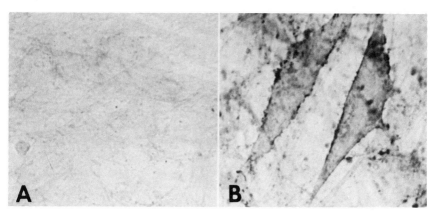

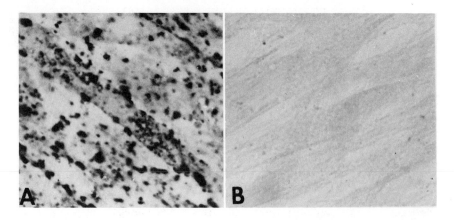

Fig. 6-12 Chick embryo cells infected with type B strain avian leukosis virus. Fixed and defatted (A) and living cells (B) were exposed to 1:10 diluted hamster antiserum to group specific (gs) antigen (devoid of antibodies to ts antigen) and, following fixation and defatting of the cells in B, both A and B were treated with rabbit serum antihamster immunoglobulin and hamster PAP (diluted 1:100) and stained for peroxidase. The group specific antigen is stained upon application to fixed and defatted (A) but not to living cells (B). The need for fixation and defatting to stain virus with gs antiserum shows that the gs antigens reside in the interior of the virus (in contrast to the ts antigens that are in the viral envelope). The failure of staining living cells shows that the hamster antiserum was devoid of anti-ts. Indistinguishable reactions were obtained with the same hamster serum anti-gs and cells infected with other types of avian leukosis virus. From the work of R. M. Dougherty, A. A. Marucci, and H. S. DiStefano, *J. Gen. Virol.,* 15:149, 1972.

rescence with ALV infected cell cultures. However, it had been carefully pointed out by G. Kelloff and P. K. Vogt that the results might be an artifact resulting from insensitivity of the method. The work of R. M. Dougherty, A. A. Marucci, and H. S. DiStefano has shown that the more sensitive unlabeled antibody-enzyme method, indeed, detects competence for making antibodies to *gs* antigens in most chickens.

Type-specific antibodies were revealed by staining of virus on the surface, and in the interior of fixed and defatted cells infected with homologous strain virus, and by complete absence of staining of cells infected with heterologous virus (Fig. 6-10). Similar type specificity was revealed upon staining of living cells, but now the stain was limited to the cell membrane (Fig. 6-11). In contrast group specific antiserum localized only virus in fixed and defatted cells but failed to localize the virus on the surface of living cells. The group specific antigens react with the interior of the viruses and are prevented from accessibility, unless the viral envelope is first disrupted by fixation and lipid extraction. The reaction is independent of the type of virus infection (Fig. 6-12). By these criteria the sera of most immunized chickens are found to contain not only type specific antibodies as expected but also group specific antibodies (Fig. 6-13). The suggestion that most or all chickens are tolerant of ALV *gs* antigens because of presence of endogenous, occult or partly expressed ALV must, therefore, be modified or discarded. These findings are the result of the increased sensitivity of the unlabeled antibody enzyme method compared to that of immunofluorescence used in earlier work.

The ease of visualization of a marker is an expression of sensitivity in light microscopy but not in electron microscopy. In light microscopy the accumulation of visualizable products as the enzyme reaction proceeds affords an amplification over the fixed amount of fluorescence obtained by fluorescent antibodies. This object is reached, however, only if the majority of antigen sites can be linked onto one or more active enzyme groups. The unlabeled antibody enzyme method assures that this occurs, since in contrast to the enzyme-conjugated antibody method none of the immunocytochemical reagents contain products that block that linkage.

Fig. 6-13 Assay of chicken serum after immunization with avian leukosis virus type B for *gs* and *ts* antibodies. Fixed and defatted cells infected (A) with type A and (B) with type B virus, and living cells infected (C) with type A and (D) with type B virus were treated with chicken antiserum, rabbit serum antichicken immunoglobulin, chicken PAP and stained for peroxidase. Staining of the heterologous infected fixed cells in A and absence of staining of the heterologous infected living cells in B reveals group specific antigen. Staining of the heterologous infected living cells in D reveals type specific antigen. The greater intensity of staining of homologous fixed (B) than of heterologous fixed cells (A) reflect the presence of both *gs* and *ts* antibodies in the serum. From the work of R. M. Dougherty, A. A. Marucci, and H. S. DiStefano, *J. Gen. Virol.*, **15**:144, 1972 (Cambridge University Press, New York, N.Y.).

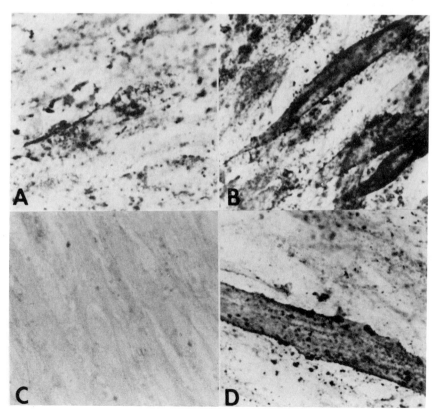

Amplification is not of the same advantage in electron microscopy as it is in light microscopy. Indeed, a single ferritin molecule is large enough to localize a specific antigen site. The enzymatic methods may yield deposits that are too heavy and may unduly mask surrounding ultrastructure. Excessive amplification in enzyme immune-electron microscopy is to be avoided by using low concentrations of substrate for peroxidase. The advantage of the unlabeled antibody enzyme method over other methods in electron microscopy rests mainly on the fact that, presumably, each reactive antigen site is being localized. No specific site is missed either by insufficient titer of antibodies or by blockage with unlabeled antibodies as is the case with the enzyme-conjugated antibody method or in some applications of the ferritin-conjugated antibody method. In contrast to the hybrid antibody method (page 99), the unlabeled antibody enzyme method does not entail significant loss of localized sites upon washing, as will be seen in our discussion on the reversibility of the immunocytochemical reaction (page 176).

SPECIFICITY

As staining control (page 53) step II is omitted, or normal serum is substituted for anti-IgG. Intrinsic peroxidase is differentiated from specifically localized antigen by the stronger reaction of the latter (Fig. 7-2) and, in post-embedding staining, by identification of the ring-shaped PAP molecules (pages 165 and 182). The high specificity of PAP itself is indicated by the fact that, in the hands of Dougherty, Marucci, and DiStefano, hamster PAP gives detectable specific staining at a 1:500 dilution, while even undiluted PAP fails to stain chicken fibroblast cultures nonspecifically.

The high sensitivity of the method may elicit, hitherto, unsuspected cross-reactions of antibodies. Even normal sera often contain some reactivity for tissue constituents localized by specific antiserum. Specific and nonspecific localization can usually be differentiated with ease, because specific sera react at high dilution, while normal sera stain only at high concentration. The reaction of normal sera may be due to natural antibodies. These "nonspecific" reactions have not been encountered with all the antigens stained so far. When found they can usually be suppressed by application prior to step I of a normal serum from the same species as the serum used in step II. Thus, it was found that normal rabbit sera stained spirochetes (*T. pallidum*) up to dilutions of 1:10. On the assumption that this staining was due to normal antibodies found in many mammalian species, the organisms were pretreated with normal sheep serum. Any sheep serum attached to the organisms would not be detectable by the method, since sheep IgG does not react with antirabbit IgG produced in sheep. The normal sheep serum blocked reaction of the spirochetes with antibodies

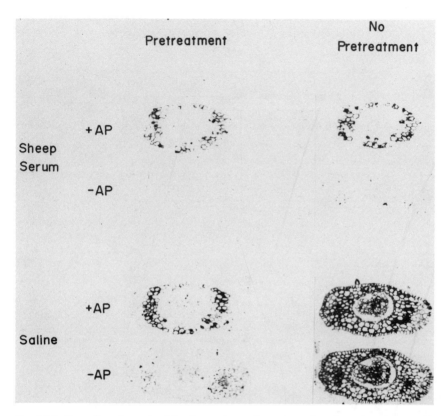

Fig. 6-14 These 8 sections of etiolated oat shoots demonstrate the effect of treatment with normal sheep serum in eliminating nonspecific staining. The sections were stained for phytochrome (chromo-receptor protein) by rabbit serum antiphytochrome (+AP), sheep serum antirabbit IgG, peroxidase-antiperoxidase complex (PAP), and cytochemistry for peroxidase. Controls were stained with normal rabbit serum (−AP), sheep serum antirabbit IgG, PAP, and cytochemistry for peroxidase. *"Pretreatment"* refers to application of sheep serum to the sections prior to the staining procedure. *"Sheep serum"* refers to *additional treatment* with normal sheep serum prior to application of sheep serum antirabbit IgG and PAP combined with dilutions of the protein-containing staining reagents in normal sheep serum. *"Saline"* refers to omission of the additional treatment. When normal sheep serum was omitted from the preincubation as well as the additional treatment, experimentally exposed and control sections were indistinguishable, indicating strong nonspecific absorption of the staining reagents to the tissue (pair of sections on the right lower part of figure). When the section was preincubated with normal sheep serum, but additional treatment was omitted, there was strong specific localization of phytochrome, but nonspecific localization was not entirely obliterated (pair of sections on left lower part of figure). When the preincubation was omitted, but normal sheep serum used in the additional treatment, specific localization did occur but, again, some nonspecific staining was evident in the control (pair of sections on right upper part of figure). Only when normal sheep serum was used in the preincubation, as well as in the additional treatment, was localization entirely specific as evident by complete absence of a picture in the control (pair of sections on left upper part of figure). From the work of Lee H. Pratt and Richard A. Coleman.

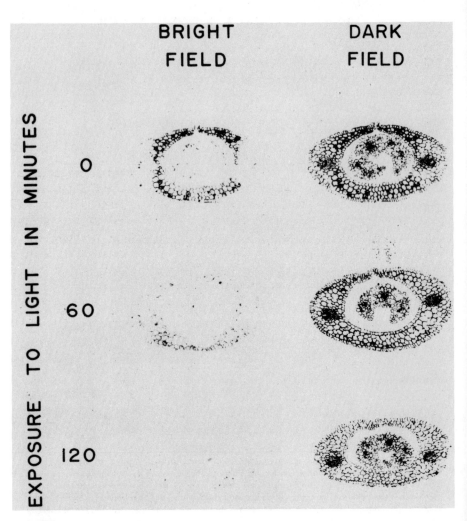

Fig. 6-15 Sections of etiolated oat shoots stained with rabbit serum antiphytochrome and the unlabeled antibody enzyme method. In bright field illumination only the phytochrome is visualized. Surrounding structure is invisible. Under dark field illumination surrounding structures become apparent, but the darkest areas are due to the strong light scattering of the product of the peroxidase reaction. Upon exposure to light, phytochrome antigen reactivity progressively disappears. X23. From the work of Lee H. Pratt and Richard A. Coleman, *Proc. Nat. Acad. Sci.*, U.S., **68**:2431, 1971.

from normal rabbit serum, and the organisms remained invisible on light microscopy. On the other hand, specific antibodies, probably by virtue of their higher concentrations and avidities, could displace the normal sheep antibodies bound on the organisms. The unlabeled antibody enzyme method was more specific than immunofluorescence in the titration of antisyphilitic antibodies even when the organisms had not been pretreated with normal sheep serum, because the titers with specific antisera were 100–1,000 times higher, while the titers with preimmunization sera were identical.

Any staining nonspecificity, at least when due to immunoglobulin-containing staining reagents, may also be prevented by addition of normal sheep serum (when sheep serum antirabbit IgG is used in step II) on the assumption that the sheep serum immunoglobulin competes with the specific staining reagents for nonspecific sites, while in itself remaining undetectable by the reagents of the method. L. H. Pratt and R. A. Coleman localized phytochrome in paraffin sections of formalin-fixed, germinated oat seeds (deparaffinized with xylene), using rabbit serum antiphytochrome (diluted 1:40), sheep serum antirabbit IgG (diluted 1:100), and rabbit PAP [diluted 1:100 (Fig. 6-14)]. To insure specificity these reagents were diluted in normal sheep serum. In addition, sections were exposed for 15 minutes in undiluted normal sheep serum immediately before application of the sheep antirabbit IgG and the PAP. The sections were washed in saline prior to exposure to normal sheep serum, but they were not washed between normal sheep serum and the succeeding specific reagents.

Phytochrome serves as a photoreceptor for a large number of photomorphogenesis responses in plants. The chromoprotein undergoes reversible absorbency changes upon exposure to light and may exert regulatory functions either via the gene mechanism or by affecting membrane permeability. Exposure to light decreases phytochrome activity *in vivo*. Using the unlabeled antibody enzyme method, exposure to light has been shown to effect disappearance of phytochrome also as an antigen (Fig. 6-15). In bright field microscopy the only structure visualized was the location of phytochrome. Nothing was seen in bright field sections in controls, or in experimentally exposed sections after 120 minutes of illumination. Hence, intrinsic peroxidase did not interfere with localization. To ascertain the relationship of specific phytochrome to nonspecific surrounding structure, dark field illumination or phase contrast microscopy can be used. In general the distribution of phytochrome was found to be highly specific regarding organs and tissues. It bore no relationship to total protein distribution or to the presence or absence of plastids or nuclei in a cell. When a cell of a given type contained phytochrome at all, it contained about the same amount as any other cell of the same type, and the phytochrome was always associated with nuclei, plastids as well as with cytoplasm. The absence of any specific organelle association of phytochrome did not yet permit a decision, whether phytochrome functioned via regulation of the gene or of membrane permeability.

In Gary oat roots almost all the phytochrome is associated with the root cap below the meristematic region and the apex of the root (Fig. 6-16). This is interesting, because the cap is a dead-end tissue that will

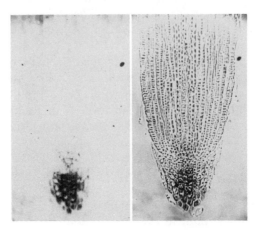

Fig. 6-16 Longitudinal sections through a young, dark grown Gary oat root, stained for phytochrome by the unlabeled antibody enzyme method. Left, bright field; right, dark field of the section. The bright field micrograph reveals about all the phytochrome in the root cap and in the apex of the root. Bright field controls give an entirely blank micrograph. The dark field micrograph reveals the surrounding structures beyond the confines of the specifically localized phytochrome. From the work of Lee H. Pratt and Richard A. Coleman.

be sloughed off. Since phytochrome is a light receptor for photomorphogenic responses, its presence in high concentration in tissue that grows in comparative darkness has been unsuspected.

Another problem of specificity is associated with the surface of blood platelets. Indeed, any white blood cell, as well as splenic plasma cells, when fixed in 4% glutaraldehyde, and exposed to peroxidase, and stained cytochemicaly without washing, reveals extensive adherence of the enzyme to the cell surface. The interior of the cell does not stain. In white blood cells washing removes the nonspecifically adherent peroxidase, but in platelets it does not. Contrary to the nonspecific adherence of free peroxidase, PAP does not adhere to platelets, at least when they are pretreated with diluted normal sheep serum. Apparently, the immunoglobulin in normal sheep serum competes for nonspecific sites with the immunoglobulin in PAP. The surface properties of PAP seem to be mainly contributed by IgG, while most of the peroxidase occupies relatively buried positions (Fig. 6-8). This is another reason for using PAP rather than the sequential application of antiperoxidase and peroxidase in the unlabeled antibody enzyme method (see also page 182).

Thrombosthenin is the actomyosin-like contractile protein that has been isolated by mild extraction from the surface, and by more extensive extraction from the interior of blood platelets. Surface thrombosthenin contributes only a minor fraction of total thrombosthenin. Thrombosthenin

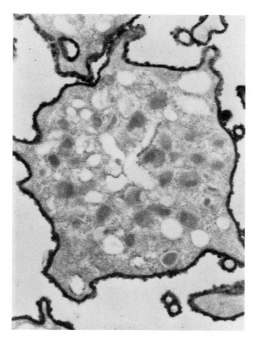

Fig. 6-17 Human platelets fixed in 4% glutaraldehyde stained for thrombosthenin by the unlabeled antibody enzyme method. Counterstained with uranyl acetate and lead citrate. The existence of surface thrombosthenin is revealed by the presence of a continuous, specific deposit along the cell membrane. X17,000. From F. M. Booyse, L. A. Sternberger, D. Zsoschke, and M. E. Rafelson, Jr., *J. Histochem Cytochem.*, **19**:540, 1971.

Fig. 6-18 Human platelets treated with pronase prior to fixation and staining for thrombosthenin by the unlabeled antibody enzyme method. No thrombosthenin is revealed on the surface of the cells. X21,600. From F. M. Booyse, L. A. Sternberger, D. Zsoschke, and M. E. Rafelson, Jr., *J. Histochem Cytochem.*, **19**:540, 1971.

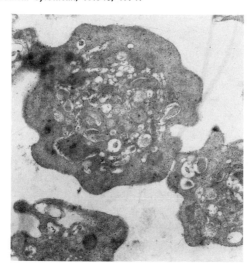

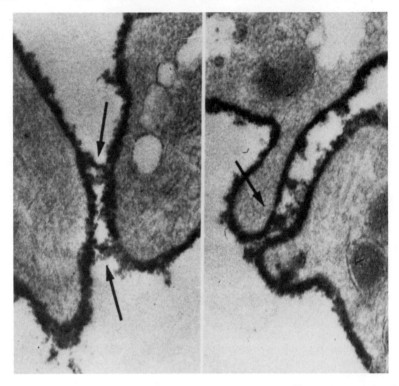

Fig. 6-19 Within 2–3 seconds after exposure of platelets with 10⁻⁷M adenosine diphosphate, surface thrombosthenin forms intracellular bridges that interlace with adjacent platelets. Unlabeled antibody enzyme method. X43,200. From the work of F. M. Booyse, T. P. Hoveke, D. Kisielski, and M. E. Rafelson, Jr., *Microcirc. Res.,* 4:179, 1972.

is involved in platelet aggregation and in clot retraction by adenosine diphosphate and thrombin. Thrombosthenin has been localized as a continuum on the surface of platelets (Fig. 6-17). Antibodies did not penetrate the interior of the cells. Cytoplasmic thrombosthenin was revealed by application of reagents to the methacrylate section (page 158).

For localization of surface thrombosthenin, the suspended platelets were treated with normal sheep serum (diluted 1:50), rabbit antithrombosthenin (diluted 1:30), sheep serum antirabbit IgG (diluted 1:5) and PAP (diluted 1:5). Platelets treated with pronase prior to staining or platelets stained with antiserum absorbed with thrombosthenin failed to reveal peroxidase reaction products (Fig. 6-18). During aggregation of platelets induced by low concentrations of adenosine diphosphate, thrombosthenin became mobilized to form intracellular bridges (Fig. 6-19). According to Booyse, the source of the surface thrombosthenin is probably cytoplasmic material "sticking" through the mosaic fluid membrane (page 103) of the platelet. When activated with adenosine diphosphate or thrombin, platelets extrude their thrombosthenin-rich cytoplasm through the cell membrane. Apparently, it is the extruded, contractile thrombosthenin and not the cell surfaces that hold agglutinated platelets together.

The unlabeled antibody enzyme method is indirect; that is, specifically localized immunoglobulin is revealed by its reaction with antiimmunoglobulin. A problem of specificity may arise if the tissue to be stained contains endogenous immunoglobulin. For instance, rabbit serum antihuman thrombosthenin was used to localize human platelet surface thrombosthenin. Sheep serum antirabbit IgG was used to reveal the rabbit antithrombosthenin. However, serum proteins are known to adhere to platelets strongly. Hence, one may suspect that the surface of platelets also possesses human immunoglobulin absorbed from plasma, which cross-reacts with rabbit immunoglobulin for sheep serum antirabbit IgG. Absorption of the sheep serum with normal human serum has abolished this possible source of nonspecificity. Difficulties may arise, however, if we were to stain an antigen in tissue from rabbit of strain A with an alloantiserum produced in rabbits

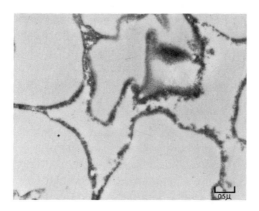

Fig. 6-20 These sheep erythrocytes (SRBC) were sensitized with a concentration of rabbit serum anti-SRBC that reacted only with a small portion of total antigen sites (discontinuous localization by the unlabeled antibody enzyme method). The cell was then reacted in sequence with guinea pig complement components 1, 4, 2, and 3. In order to block the anti-SRBC against staining by the unlabeled antibody enzyme method, the cell was treated with sheep FAb anti-rabbit IgG prior to localization of the third complement component (C3) with rabbit serum antiguinea pig C3. Staining by sheep serum antirabbit IgG and PAP and cyochemistry for peroxidase reveals localization of C3 as a continuum over the cells. From the work of L. A. Sternberger.

of strain B. The sheep antirabbit IgG would react with both the endogenous immunoglobulin of strain A as well as with the bound immunoglobulin of strain B. To limit reaction of the sheep antirabbit IgG to strain B immunoglobulin, the reaction of endogenous immunoglobulin can conceivably be blocked by pretreatment with FAb from sheep IgG antirabbit IgG. The FAb will react with the endogenous immunoglobulin of strain A, but being monovalent, will not be able to react with subsequently applied PAP. The effectiveness of this approach is illustrated by the localization of guinea pig complement component 3 (C3) with rabbit antiguinea pig C3 on sheep erythrocytes (SRBC) sensitized with rabbit anti-SRBC. Since diluted anti-SRBC was used for sensitization, localization of the antibody was limited to discrete sites [similar to Figs. 7-1 (d) and 3-10]. However, after reaction with complement components 1, 4, 2, and 3, localization of rabbit anti-C3 was continuous (Fig. 6-20). In order to insure that the sheep antirabbit immunoglobulin would react only with the rabbit anti-C3 and not with the rabbit-SRBC, sheep FAb anti-IgG was applied to EA1, 4, 2a, 3b (page 6) before staining with anti-C3 and the unlabeled antibody enzyme method. The entire staining was abolished when the rabbit anti-C3 had been absorbed with C3. This demonstrates that the FAb had effectively blocked the sites of attachment of rabbit anti-SRBC against staining by the unlabeled antibody enzyme method.

POST-EMBEDDING STAINING

When PAP is applied to ultrathin Epon or methacrylate sections, the entire surface becomes heavily stained by DAB and hydrogen peroxide because of extensive nonspecific adsorption of PAP. This nonspecific adsorption is abolished if the section is pretreated with diluted normal sheep serum. Similarly, normal rabbit serum followed by sheep serum antirabbit IgG and PAP gives strong nonspecific staining. This staining is due to nonspecific adsorption of the normal rabbit serum, since it disappears when the sheep serum antirabbit IgG is omitted. Again the nonspecific adsorption of normal rabbit serum can be blocked by pretreatment with normal sheep serum. When sheep serum antirabbit IgG is applied first and followed by PAP, there is no staining. Apparently, the antirabbit IgG *is* adsorbed nonspecifically, since otherwise, the PAP would have been adsorbed nonspecifically, resulting in staining. The adsorption of antirabbit IgG on the section seems to be so strong as to distort or hinder its specific antibody combining sites and to prevent, thereby, binding with PAP. The observations suggest that any protein is adsorbed to electron microscopy sections nonspecifically, and that the adsorption is strong enough to prevent adsorption of a subsequently applied protein even if the section is being washed. Serum immunoglobulins of one species prevent the adsorption of immunoglobulins of another species but not necessarily that of proteins with different net charges, such as ferritin, or free peroxidase, or immunoglobulins conjugated with polar or hydrophobic substituents. These considerations suggest for the unlabeled antibody enzyme method the pretreatment of thin sections with dilute, normal serum of the same species that donates the anti-IgG. This serum, of course, will fail to react with the anti-IgG and, thus, will not be detected by PAP.

For post-embedding staining, silver or light gold Araladite or Epon sections are placed on nickel grids (150 mesh, formvar coated; or 300 mesh, uncoated). The sections are etched by floating for three minutes on drops of a 5% aqueous solution of hydrogen peroxide on glass slides. The sections are "jet washed" by a spray of saline from a plastic spray bottle and "blotted" by holding them edgewise onto filter paper. The immunologic reagents are applied by floating the sections on drops of solution in shallow depressions in paraffin or on flat dental wax in covered Petri dishes, using the following sequence: normal serum of species B (page 129) diluted 1:30 in saline, for five minutes at room temperature, followed by blotting, but not by washing; primary antiserum (page 129) for five minutes at room temperature, or up to 48 hours at 2–5° (permitting the dishes to reequilibriate to room temperature for the last 1–2 hours), followed by jet washing in buffer and blotting; normal serum of species B, diluted 1:30 in buffer, for five minutes at room temperature, followed by blotting, but not by washing; antiserum of species B reactive with IgG of the species that has supplied the primary antiserum, diluted 1:10 in buffer, for five minutes at room temperature, followed by jet washing in buffer and blotting; normal serum of species B, diluted 1:30 in buffer, for five minutes at room temperature, followed by blotting, but not by washing; PAP, diluted 1:50 in buffer containing 1% of normal serum of species B, for five minutes at room temperature, followed by jet washing is 0.05 M Tris buffer, pH 7.6, but not by blotting. The grids, held by forceps, are then immersed for three minutes at room temperature into a beaker containing a freshly prepared solution of 0.0125% diaminobenzidine tetrahydrochloride and 0.0025% hydrogen peroxide in 0.05 M Tris buffer, pH 7.6. This solution is kept under agitation over a magnetic stirrer at 50–80 rpm. The grids are rapidly transferred for about 30 seconds to another beaker containing water, also kept under agitation. Following removal from the water, the sections are jet washed in water, blotted, and placed on filter paper. The sections are then floated on a 4% solution of aqueous osmium tetroxide in porcelain depression dishes for 10–25 minutes and again washed in water. Nickel or gold grids are necessary to avoid reaction of the grid bars with osmium. During the staining procedure up to (but not including) the osmium step, the grids are never allowed to dry completely.

All solutions are prepared from distilled, deionized, Millipore-filtered water. Any commonly used buffer, pH 7.2–7.6, made isotonic by dilution in normal saline, is satisfactory for the stages preceding the staining with diaminobenzidine. However, the diaminobenzidine must be dissolved in 0.05 M Tris buffer, pH 7.6. All undiluted sera are stored at or below −20°C after freezing in dry ice and acetone. They are thawed in a 37°C water bath. All undiluted sera are Millipore filtered either before or after storage. The normal sera are decomplemented in a water bath at 56°C for 30 minutes.

Most of the work on post-embedding staining, including that which first established its sensitivity, has been done with primary antisera applied for 2–5 minutes. However, Gwen Moriarty discovered that, especially when highly diluted primary antisera are employed, sensitivity can be increased by another factor of 1,000 if exposure to primary antiserum is prolonged to 48 hours. This prolonged exposure does not induce nonspecific background staining, but will reveal antibodies, hitherto unsuspected by less sensitive immunologic methods and will require more extensive immunocytochemical controls for specificity (page 52).

Buffers containing 1% of normal serum of species B are used for dilution of primary antiserum at, or above, 1,000 fold. At lesser dilutions it is necessary to increase the concentration of normal serum to not less than 10 fold that of the primary antiserum; *i.e.,* a 1:100 dilution of primary antiserum should be used in buffer containing 10% of normal serum. For antihormone sera, buffers containing 0.25% human serum albumin are substituted for those containing 1% normal serum of species B, because the hormone contents of normal serum inhibit staining to a small extent, at least when analyzed quantitatively (page 181). This may provide a sensitive hormone assay.

The details of the above staining sequence were arrived at by quantitative comparison of several alternatives in the laboratories of Ludwig Sternberger and Gwen Moriarty. The sequence assures maximum sensitivity and clean preparations.

Choice of fixation depends on the particular antigen examined. 2.5% glutaraldehyde at room temperature has been the fixative of choice for corticotropin, melanocyte-stimulating hormone, thrombosthenin, and lysozyme. Formaldehyde-picric acid is the preferred fixative for prolactin, follicle-stimulating hormone and luteinizing hormone. In general free cells should be fixed for only 5 to 10 minutes, while pieces of tissue (about 1 mm^3) require fixation for 1–3 hours. Paraformaldehyde fixation destroys thrombosthenin and extracts intermediate lobe corticotropin, although it does preserve for post-embedding staining the antigenic reactivity of anterior lobe corticotropin, pneumococcal polysaccharide, and λ-phage. With any new antigen, glutaraldehyde fixation should be attempted first because of the superior preservation of structure. Sometimes, satisfactory fixation can be obtained with as little as 0.125% glutaraldehyde in 5% sucrose at room temperature for three hours.

Gwen Moriarty and N. S. Halmi studied the formation and distribution of corticotropin (ACTH) in the anterior and intermediate lobes of the pituitary, using dilutions of rabbit antiserum to the 17–39 peptide of ACTH

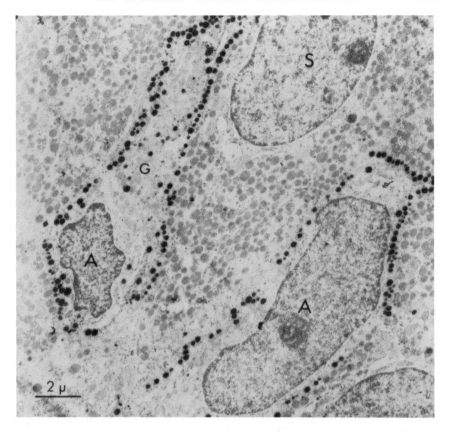

Fig. 6-21 Anterior lobe of rat pituitary, glutaraldehyde fixation, stained on the araldite section with anti-$\beta_p{}^{17-39}$ corticotropin (ACTH), diluted 1:20, and the unlabeled antibody enzyme method. The ACTH cell (A) is stellate possessing peripherally arranged granules of homogenous size that contain specific reaction product. Cell processes often reach the wall of a capillary. Granules in the Golgi complex (G) are always stained. S, thyrotrope. (The anti-ACTH used in Figs. 6-21 to 6-28 bound, when undiluted, 17% of 5 pg of added ^{125}I-ACTH per ml. At a dilution of 1:30, binding was 3%.) From the work of G. C. Moriarty and N. S. Halmi, *J. Histochem. Cytochem.,* **20**:590, 1972.

$(\beta_p{}^{17-39})$ and the unlabeled antibody enzyme method on Araldite sections. The $\beta_p{}^{17-39}$ ACTH, unlike the whole ACTH molecule, possesses no cross-reactivity with melanocyte-stimulating hormone that is also secreted in the intermediate lobe.

In the anterior lobe specific staining characterizes the ACTH cell as a stellate cell amidst gonadotropic, thyrotropic, and growth hormone cells (Fig. 6-21). The granules are arranged peripherally, usually in a single row. Often a process of the cell makes direct contact with the wall of a capillary. Granules in the Golgi region stain also. Following adrenalectomy,

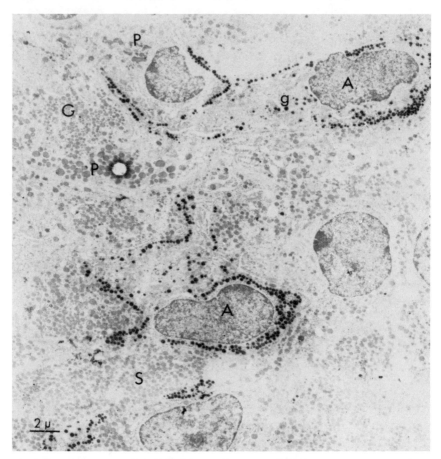

Fig. 6-22 Anterior lobe of rat pituitary 21 days after adrenalectomy, stained on the araldite section with anti-β_p^{17-39} ACTH, diluted 1:20, and the unlabeled antibody enzyme method. In the rebound after adrenalectomy, the ACTH cells (A) are increased in number and contain a larger amount of specifically staining granules. The cells remain stellate, and the Golgi complex (g) contains strongly staining granules. From the work of G. C. Moriarty and N. S. Halmi, J. Histochem. Cytochem., 20:590, 1972.

the number of specifically stained granules diminishes, and the intensity of their staining decreases. Three weeks after adrenalectomy at the time when physiologic measurements indicate a rebound of ACTH contents to levels three times those of normal tissue, the stained cells are more numerous (Fig. 6-22) and contain a larger number of granules. However, the characteristic stellate shape and the peripheral arrangement of the granules is maintained. The Golgi region contains several granules that stain very strongly. Apparently, the Golgi complex of the anterior lobe ACTH cell

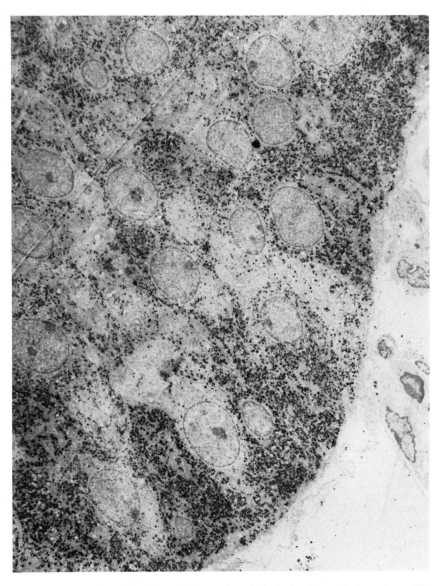

Fig. 6-23 Intermediate lobe of rat pituitary, glutaraldehyde fixation, stained on the araldite section with anti-$\beta_{\mathrm{P}}^{17-39}$ ACTH, diluted 1:20, and the unlabeled antibody enzyme method. Each parenchymal cell contains a large number of deeply stained granules. The granules gather towards one pole of the cell. X4,500. From the work of G. C. Moriarty and N. S. Halmi.

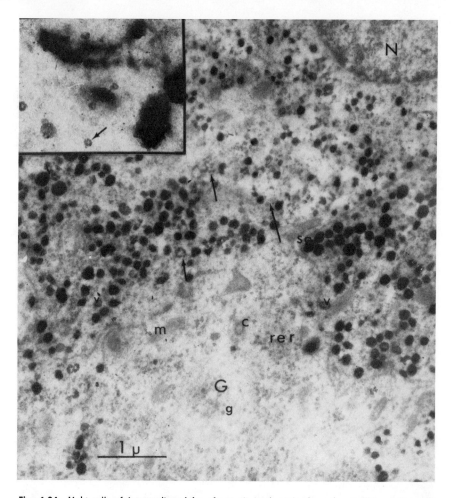

Fig. 6-24 Light cells of intermediate lobe of rat pituitary, stained on the araldite section with anti-$\beta_P{}^{17-39}$ ACTH, diluted 1:200, and the unlabeled antibody enzyme method. Secretory granules (sg) and vesicles are stained. Often only the rim of the vesicles (V) stain. The membranous structures (arrows) may be rough endoplasmic reticulum. The Golgi region (G), the granules in the Golgi region (g), and the mitochondria (m) are free of reaction product. C, centriole. X20,000. Inset shows a secretory granule and an irregularly shaped vesicle. The stain on the vesicle outlines membranes as clumps of varying size. The cytoplasm in regions near the secretory granules often reveals single molecules of peroxidase-antiperoxidase complex (PAP) (arrows). They average 31 nm in diameter and are either ring, pentagon, or U-shaped. Inset 60,500. From the work of G. C. Moriarty and N. S. Halmi, *Z. Zellforsch.*, **132**:1, 1972 (Springer Verlag, Berlin-Heidelberg-New York).

functions as in many other secretory cells as a collecting apparatus for the secreted product.

The parenchymal cells of the intermediate lobe consist of the so-called light cells and the less numerous dark cells. Both these cell types stain alike for ACTH (Fig. 6-23). Most of the ACTH is found in pleomorphic secretion granules, but some stain is seen on membranes of vesicles and apparently on endoplasmic reticulum (Fig. 6-24). The stain on secretion granules is too intense to permit discrimination of individual PAP molecules in this location. However, in cytoplasmic areas close to the secretion granules individual PAP molecules are seen. Apparently, the concentration of ACTH in this location is so low that antigen sites are dispersed and the attached PAP well separated (see also page 173). No ACTH is found on mitochondria and in nuclei, and there is a striking absence of ACTH from some granules in the Golgi zone.

Dark cells have fewer secretory granules than light cells (Fig. 6-25). However, their staining pattern is identical, and again the Golgi structures are unstained, and the cisternae of the endoplasmic reticulum are empty.

In dark as well as light cells, intensity of staining on the vesicles varies, while staining of the granules is always intense. The attachment of ribosomes to the membranes of some of the vesicles suggests that the vesicles may be part of the endoplasmic reticulum.

Progressive dilution of anti-$\beta_p{}^{17-39}$ ACTH permits some quantitation of the relative amounts of ACTH found in different regions. Antiserum has to be diluted extensively to yield partial staining over the secretion granules.

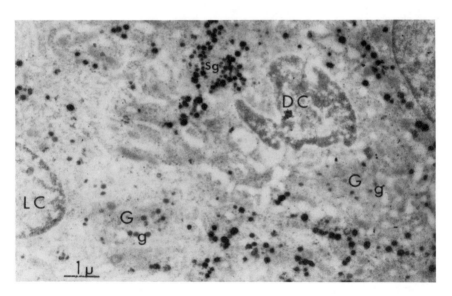

Fig. 6-25 A dark cell (DC) next to light cells (LC), stained on the araldite section with anti-$\beta_p{}^{17-39}$ ACTH, diluted 1:20, and the unlabeled antibody enzyme method. The secretory granules (Sg) of the dark cell stain as those of the light cell. The Golgi region (G) of the light as well as the dark cell is unstained and the rough endoplasmic reticulum is diluted and unstained. g, Golgi complex granules. From the work of G. C. Moriarty and N. S. Halmi, Z. Zellforsch., 132:1, 1972 (Springer Verlag, Berlin-Heidelberg-New York).

The staining intensity in Fig. 6-26 is considered to be the limiting titer of the antiserum (lowest concentration that gives definite staining; 1:2,000 after application for two to three minutes in Fig. 6-26). In only 25% of granules is the stain intense enough to completely blacken the structure, while in the remainder of granules staining is not uniform. At times only the rim of secretion granules and vesicles is stained, apparently, indicating higher concentrations of antigen at the periphery. Occasional clumps of the characteristic ring-shaped or pentagonal PAP molecules seen at high dilution of antiserum on vesicular membranes may identify ACTH on endoplasmic reticulum.

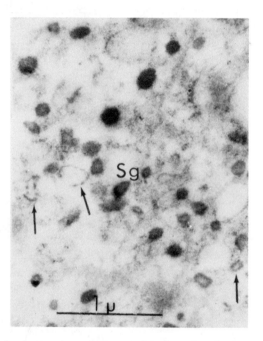

Fig. 6-26 Light cell stained on the Araldite section with anti-$\beta_p{}^{17-39}$ ACTH, diluted 1:2,000, and the unlabeled antibody enzyme method. Reaction product is on rough endoplasmic reticulum (arrows). In the secretory granules (Sg) it is the rim that stains most intensely at this dilution. This is considered the maximal dilution of the anti-$\beta_p{}^{17-39}$ ACTH at which staining is obtainable upon two to three minutes exposure. Much higher dilutions give positive staining upon 48 hours exposure. From the work of G. C. Moriarty and N. S. Halmi, *Z. Zellforsch.*, **132**:1, 1972 (Springer Verlag, Berlin-Heidelberg-New York).

Fairly high concentrations of normal serum (1–100 in Fig. 6-27) also yield minimal staining for ACTH. This is probably the effect of normal antibodies in serum, since replacement of anti-$\beta_p{}^{17-39}$ ACTH with buffer or omission of the antirabbit IgG after application of anti-$\beta_p{}^{17-39}$ ACTH in the otherwise complete staining procedure yields entirely negative micrographs.

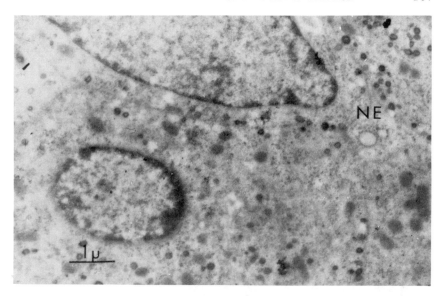

Fig. 6-27 Light cells stained on the araldite section with normal rabbit serum, diluted 1:100, and the unlabeled antibody enzyme method. There is slight deposition of reaction product along the rim of some of the secretory granules. NE, nerve endings. From the work of G. C. Moriarty, and N. S. Halmi, Z. *Zellforsch.*, **132**:1, 1972 (Springer Verlag, Berlin-Heidelberg-New York).

Portions of the anterior lobe that interdigitate with the intermediate lobe afford opportunity to compare ACTH in both locations on the same section (Fig. 6-28). In the anterior lobe only a small proportion of cells are ACTH cells, while in the intermediate lobe all cells contain specifically staining granules except for the cuboidal or flattened epithelial cells bordering the lobules. In the anterior lobe ACTH granules are confined to the periphery of the characteristic stellate cell that is often in contact with capillaries of the highly vascularized lobe. In the intermediate lobe, which may be more under neural than hormonal control, vascularization is poor, and the secretion granules bear no relation to capillaries. The granules fill a major portion of at least one pole of the cellular cytoplasm. The concentration per granule is also higher in the intermediate than in the anterior lobe. The same serum that gives minimal staining at a 1:2,000 concentration in the intermediate lobe yields minimal staining at a 1:500 concentration in the anterior lobe. In the anterior lobe the granules are of uniform size, and each granule itself stains uniformly. In the intermediate lobe the granules are heterogeneous in size, and the concentration of ACTH within individual granules is not uniform. While the Golgi zone contains ACTH in the anterior lobe, it is strikingly free of ACTH in the intermediate lobe. Immunocytochemical evidence suggests that in the anterior lobe the sequence of ACTH formation resembles that of most other protein-secreting

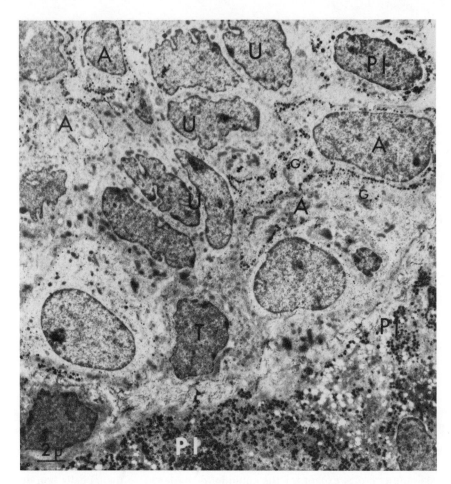

Fig. 6-28 Area from the rostral part of the adenohypophysis containing ACTH cells from the anterior lobe interdigitating with cells from the intermediate lobe. The gland is from a rat that had been adrenalectomized and injected with cortisol. Glutaraldehyde fixation. Stained on the section with anti-β_P^{17-39} ACTH, diluted 1:100, and the unlabeled antibody enzyme method. Counterstained with uranyl acetate and lead citrate. The anterior lobe ACTH cell (A) is stellate and has peripherally arranged granules of 214 nm maximum diameter that contain immunospecific reaction product. The Golgi complex (G) is strongly stained. Another ACTH cell contains secretory granules that are smaller, but still they are of rather uniform size with 100 nm maximum diameter. The intermediate lobe (P1) presents "light cells" which all contain numerous strongly staining secretory granules. T, thyrotrope. U, undifferentiated cell. From G. C. Moriarty and N. S. Halmi, *Z. Zellforsch.*, **132**:1, 1972 (Springer Verlag, Berlin-Heidelberg-New York).

cells. In the intermediate lobe the striking absence of ACTH from the Golgi region and from the channels of the endoplasmic reticulum of those areas of the cell in which there are few secretory granules, and the presence of ACTH on vesicles, membranes, and ribosomes that are in proximity to the ACTH-containing granules suggest that ACTH is produced, condensed, and packaged only in certain regions of the cell. If collection of protein is the function of the Golgi apparatus and of the channels of the endoplasmic reticulum, then in the cells of the intermediate lobe these areas still represent structures in search of a specific protein.

The work of Stan Erlandsen on post-embedding staining of intestinal Paneth cells (Fig. 6-9c) suggests a pathway of lysozyme formation and action in this location. Evidently newly formed lysozyme appearing in the Golgi region is stored in the granules of the Paneth cells. The stored material is exocytosed and bound to the microvillar border of adjacent cells. Conceivably, the lysozyme so distributed over the luminal surface of the intestine plays a role in the defense against bacterial invasion.

The use of peroxidase or any other enzyme that is available in pure form and can be stained histochemically affords an amplification to the detection of antibodies. This amplification gives the unlabeled antibody enzyme method a sensitivity 100–1,000 times that of immunofluorescence and 1,000 times that of radioimmunoassay. However, the enzymatic detector alone is not responsible for this increase in sensitivity as the enzyme-*conjugated* antibody method is only equally as sensitive as immunofluorescence. Another reason for the high sensitivity of the unlabeled antibody enzyme method is staining efficiency. The use of only unlabeled antibodies in attaching the enzyme specifically to the tissue antigen site assures that each antigen site is linked to at least one, but in general to a number of active enzyme molecules. Only steric hindrance could prevent detection of each antigen site when staining is intense and antigen closely packed. However, when staining is weak and antigen distribution sparse, no reagent interferes with localization of practically each antigen site by cytochemically reacting enzyme.

In high resolution electron microscopy the sensitivity sought is detection of a single molecule. The ferritin-labeled antibody method and certainly the hybrid antibody method accomplishes this degree of sensitivity, since each individual ferritin molecule can be discerned. The unlabeled antibody enzyme method also detects single antibody molecules as will be shown in the next chapter on molecular immunocytochemistry. The high sensitivity of the unlabeled antibody enzyme method permits use of dilute reagents.

Reversibility of the antigen antibody reaction, that is dissociation of bound antibody during washing, becomes an important factor in high resolution electron immunocytochemistry. For single molecule detection, dissociation during washing may make the difference between a positive or negative stain for this molecule. Reversibility has been studied for the unlabeled antibody enzyme method (page 176).

Both the hybrid antibody ferritin and the unlabeled antibody enzyme methods are free of the most important contributors to nonspecificity, namely increased polarity and hydrophobicity of reagents as a result of labeling procedures. In both methods the use of only native proteins insures that their surface properties do not differ drastically from those of tissue proteins. In addition preparation of purified PAP in the unlabeled antibody enzyme method is a high yield procedure. Consequently, the antisera against the tissue constituents under investigation can be used in higher dilutions than in other methods. The effect of nonspecifically reacting serum constituents, if any, is thereby minimized.

Single molecule sensitivity, high specificity, and low reversibility suggest the unlabeled antibody enzyme method for use in quantitative and molecular immunocytochemistry discussed in the next chapter.

REFERENCES

Booyse, F. M. and Rafelson, M. E., Jr. Human platelet contractile proteins: location, properties, and function. *Ser. Haemat.*, 4:152, 1971.

Booyse, F. M., Sternberger, L. A., Zschocke, D., and Rafelson, M. E. Jr. Ultrastructural localization of contractile protein (thrombosthenin) in human platelets using an unlabeled antibody peroxidase staining technique. *J. Histochem. Cytochem.*, 19:540, 1971.

Dougherty, R. M., Marucci, A. A., and DiStefano, H. S. Application of immunohistochemistry to the study of avian leukosis virus. *J. Gen. Virol.*, 15:149, 1972.

Kelloff, G. and Vogt, P. K. Localization of avian tumor virus group specific antigen in cell and virus. *Virology*, 29:377, 1966.

Kuettner, K. E., Eisenstein, R., Soble, L. W., and Arsenis, C. Lysozyme in epiphyseal cartilage. IV. Embryonic chick cartilage lysozyme—its localization and partial characterization. *J. Cell Biol.*, 49:450, 1971.

Moriarty, G. C. Adenohypophysis: Ultrastructural cytomchemistry (a review). *J. Histochem. Cytochem.*, 21:855, 1973.

Moriarty, G. C. and Halmi, N. S. Adrenocorticotropin production by the intermediate lobe of the rat pituitary: An electron microscopic immunocytochemical study. *Z. Zellforsch.*, 132:1, 1972.

Moriarty, G. C. and Halmi, N. S. Electron microscopic localization of the adrenocorticotropin-producing cell with the use of unlabeled antibody and the peroxidase-antiperoxidase complex. *J. Histochem. Cytochem.*, 20:590, 1972.

Moriarty, G. C., Moriarty, C. M., and Sternberger, L. A. Ultrastructural immunocytochemistry by unlabeled antibodies and the peroxidase-antiperoxidase complex (PAP). A technique more sensitive than radioimmunoassay. *J. Histochem. Cytochem.*, 21:825, 1973.

Pratt, L. H. and Coleman, R. A. Immunocytochemical localization of phytochrome. *Proc. Nat. Acad. Sci.*, U.S., 68:2431, 1971.

Sternberger, L. A. Enzyme immunohistochemistry. In "Electron Microscopy of Enzymes: Principles and Methods." Vol. I, M. A. Hayat (ed.). Von Nostrand Reinhold Co., New York, 1973.

Sternberger, L. A. Some new developments in immunocytochemistry. *Mikroskopie*, 25:346, 1969.

Sternberger, L. A. The unlabeled antibody-peroxidase and the quantitative immunouranium methods in light and electron immunohistochemistry. *Tech. Biochem Biophys. Morphol.*, 1:67, 1972.

Sternberger, L. A., Hardy, P. H., Jr., Cuculis, J. J., and Meyer, H. G. The unlabeled antibody-enzyme method of immunohistochemistry. Preparation and properties of soluble antigen-antibody complex (horseradish peroxidase-antihorseradish peroxidase) and its use in identification of spirochetes. *J. Histochem. Cytochem.*, 18:315, 1970.

Chapter 7

Molecular Immunocytochemistry

The concentration of a chemical compound is the quantitative expression of the number of molecules in a defined space. Uniform distribution of molecules permits measurement of concentration in a small aliquot of the total sample. For instance, if we want to know the concentration of circulating fibrinogen we are justified in drawing a small blood sample, clotting a defined amount of plasma, and measuring the protein contents of the washed clot. We are still justified to apply similar rationale for measurement of concentrations at the cytochemical level seen in the light microscope. We can stain smears of platelets with antiplatelet serum and fluorescein-conjugated anti-IgG and scan the preparation with a fluorescent microscope equipped with a light intensity recorder, averaging the optical densities recorded and comparing the values for afibrinogenemic and normal platelets. By recording a large number of areas from many representative platelets, we will have randomized unevenness of distribution of fibrinogen within individual platelets and, hence, the ratio of average optical densities of afibrinogenemic and normal platelets will tell us whether the amount of fibrinogen in afibrinogenemic platelets is less than in normal platelets or not. Thus, we still can express amounts of fibrinogen in terms of concentration. If we increase by electron microscopy the resolution to a level at which the confines of single molecules can be discerned, our recorder should take advantage of this resolution by measuring areas not larger than the immunocytochemical deposits resulting from reaction with a single molecule. In such an area optical density measurements of electron opacity, under ideal circumstances, will either be positive or negative, depending upon the presence or absence of a specifically stained molecule. There will be no intermediate values, since no fractional molecules can be seen. Hence, it is neither possible nor desirable to assign an optical density value to a cytochemical area at high resolution. Instead, one can enumerate the number of molecules that are found in a specific structure such as a membrane of endoplasmic reticulum. Results will have to be expressed in terms of number of molecules per segment of a specific membrane rather than in terms of concentration per electron beam area. Therefore, we call this approach "molecular immunocytochemistry." We contrast it with "quantitative immunocytochemistry," which depends on recording of optical densities of a subcellular structure rather than enumeration of molecules contained in it.

Molecular immunocytochemistry is only possible if each deposit is an amplified site of a single antigen molecule. The deposit is always larger than the antigen molecule. Hence, deposits coalesce when antigen molecules are closely packed, thus, preventing enumeration. Only if antigen-bearing molecules are widely separated will enumeration of spots correspond to number of molecules.

Surface antigens of sheep erythrocytes (SRBC) offer a model for establishing the validity of this approach to quantitative staining immunocytochemistry. When the cells are reacted with increasing amounts of ^{125}I-labeled rabbit IgG_2 anti-SRBC, a saturation concentration is reached beyond which the number of cell-bound counts does not increase. From the specific radioactivity of the IgG_2 used, the number of SRBC, and their known surface area, the number of molecues of anti-SRBC bound per cell at saturation is found to be 2,600,000.

Addition to SRBC of 1/50th or 1/500th of the saturation concentration of anti-SRBC and staining by the unlabeled antibody enzyme method leads to a continuous deposit of reaction product on the cell [Fig. 7-1 (a) and (b)]. The agglutination titer of the anti-SRBC used was 1/5,000th the saturation concentration; that is, at this dilution some cells were still visibly agglutinated, but most of them remained unagglutinated. Nevertheless, enzymatic staining reveals only partial discontinuity of staining on the cell surface [Fig. 7-1 (c)]. However, most of the staining is still seen in patches, and enumeration of single sites is impossible. The relative paucity of unreacted antigen-bearing areas suggests that antibody must be in considerable excess to facilitate extensive agglutination of cells. Apparently, both antigen-binding sites of IgG antibody attach preferentially to adjacent antigen sites on a single cell rather than by cross-linking two cells.

Only at higher dilutions do the deposits become discrete. With increasing dilution the chance increases that each deposit represents a single, bound anti-SRBC molecule rather than a group of closely packed molecules. Hence, enumeration of sites is only possible with high concentrations of antibodies when the cell antigen concentration is low or, as in the present artificial model, with low concentrations of antibody when the cell antigen concentration is high. The number of sites per cell reacted at 1/50,000th the saturation concentration of anti-SRBC is around 1,000 and at 1/500,000th around 100 [Fig. 7-1 (d) and (e)].

If the concentration of diaminobenzidine tetrahydrochloride is 0.05% and that of hydrogen peroxide 0.01%, the size of discrete spots on the cell

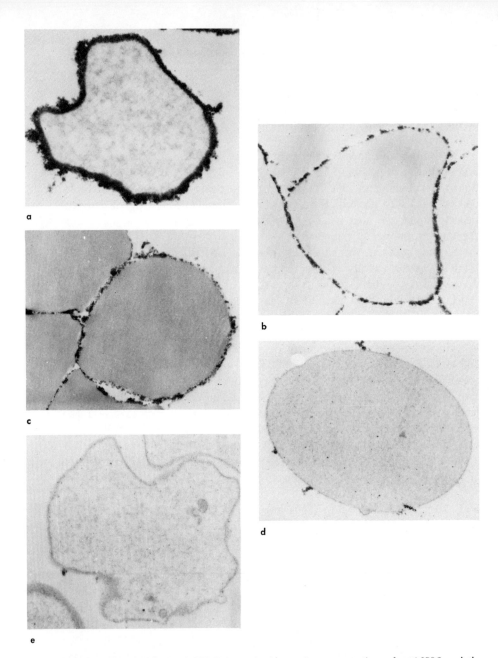

Fig. 7-1 Sheep erythrocytes (SRBC) reacted with varying concentrations of anti-SRBC and the unlabeled antibody enzyme method and embedded after staining in low viscosity epon. 100 nm thick sections. (a) concentration of anti-SRBC 1/50 of the saturation level. (b) 1/500 of the saturation level. (c) 1/5,000 of the saturation level. (d) 1/50,000 of the saturation level. (e) 1/500,000 of the saturation level. Only at concentrations of 1/50,000 the saturation level and lower are the deposits sufficiently separated to permit their enumeration as representing single anti-SRBC molecules. The intensity of specific deposits in the unlabeled antibody enzyme method by far exceeds that of the intrinsic peroxidatic activity in the interior of the erythrocytes. From the work of L. A. Sternberger.

174

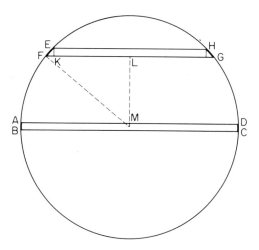

Fig. 7-2 An equatorial section (ABCD) and an off-center section (EFGH) of finite and equal thickness (AB=EK=d) through an idealized round cell with radius, r. The cell membrane antigen sites seen in electron microscopy of an equatorial section are contributed by an area of the cell membrane defined by a 360° rotation around the axis LM of a band of width AB, which is $2\pi rd$ (assuming that the section thickness is small relative to the diameter of the cell). The cell membrane antigen sites seen on an off-center section are defined by a 360° rotation around the axis LM of a band with a width EF. Since < FEK = < FMA = α and EF = $d/\cos\alpha$, and since FL = $r\cos\alpha$, the area viewed in the off-center section is $2\pi(EF)(LF) = 2\pi(r\cos\alpha)(d/\cos\alpha)$ = $2\pi rd$ which is equal to the area viewed on the equatorial section.

surface is variable as in Fig. 7-1 (c) and (d). A lesser concentration of these reagents is preferable, as it decreases the size of individual spots and the variance of size of one spot to another without affecting the total number of spots.

If we assume that a cell approximates the shape of a sphere, it does not matter whether an electron microscopy section is equatorial [Fig. 7-2 (ABCD)] or off-center (EFGH). In off-center sections the cell membrane is cut at an angle and is partially viewed on its face. As a consequence the membrane appears thicker, and the number of deposits seen per unit length increases. However, the increase in number of deposits cancels with the decrease of circumference of the membrane.

In the preceding chapters we have evaluated the validity of immuno-cytochemical methods by their sensitivities and specificities. A method appeared useful if the specific localization was intense relative to non-specific localization. The criteria were entirely histologic. To evaluate an immunocytochemical method in more objective terms, we should raise the question whether a single spot viewed histologically does indeed represent a single antigenic determinant or its specific antibody measured by independent means.

When ^{125}I-labeled IgG$_2$ anti-SRBC is used in the unlabeled antibody enzyme method, and radioactivity determinations are made *after* completion of the staining sequence, the number of spots counted by electron microscopy equals the number of anti-IgG$_2$ molecules measured by radioactivity at any concentration of anti-IgG$_2$ applied at which discrete spots can be enumerated electron microscopically. In addition the number of spots counted after application of varying concentrations of IgG$_2$ within the discrete spot range bears a linear relationship to the total peroxidase activity of SRBC ghosts obtained from cells that have been brought through the PAP step. These criteria provide two independent lines of evidence for the validity of observed cytochemical localization by the unlabeled antibody enzyme method. The evidence permits the conclusion, that if spots of opacity are well separated in an electron microscopic field, each spot represents, indeed, the amplified deposit of a single antigen determinant. Thus, the individual sites seen by Gwen Moriarty and N. S. Halmi on the endoplasmic reticulum near the ACTH secretory granules (Fig. 6-24) correspond, indeed, to single molecules of ACTH, save for one reservation.

In fact the spots represent only the reacted antigen sites at the end of the immunocytochemical staining procedure. This number may be less than those reacted initially, because losses may have occurred during incubation and washings. This is why avidity considerations are so important in critical immunocytochemistry. In the next section we shall evaluate the dissociation of reacted antibodies from cells during immunocytochemical staining to determine what correction factors, if any, are necessary for quantitation by the unlabeled antibody enzyme method in absolute terms.

REVERSIBILITY OF THE IMMUNOCYTOCHEMICAL REACTION

The avidities of antibodies, at least in the case of antibodies from late hyperimmune sera, are usually high enough that only a fraction of bound antibody is expected to be lost during the washing in immunocytochemical reactions. However, dissociation does occur and is promoted by increase in wash volume and temperature. Indeed, purified antibody can be obtained in fair yields by reacting sheep erythrocytes (SRBC) with anti-SRBC, washing the agglutinated cells in the cold, and eluting antibody from the cells by repeated treatments with large volumes of neutral buffer at 37°.

In most qualitative immunocytochemical reactions the dissociation of antibody during washing is a negligible factor, for even as much as 50% loss of bound antibody would not materially alter the observations. In quantitative enumeration of antibody binding sites, however, reversibility cannot be ignored.

In the localization of antigen sites on the SRBC model discussed above, each protein reagent of the unlabeled antibody enzyme method was applied to the cells in suspension for 10 minutes at 25°. The cells were then washed three times at 2°. At this temperature dissociation is known to be negligible. After washing the cells were incubated in the next reagent of the stepwise procedure. During this incubation, dissociation of each of the precedingly applied reagents could occur. In fact, during each step of the staining procedure, about 0.2% of the anti-SRBC is lost (Table 7-1, lines 1-3, Figs. 7-3

Table 7-1

Dissociation of reagents during staining by the unlabeled antibody enzyme method

	Test cells added to treated cells	Step of admixture of test cells	Antibody disso- ciation measured	Number of molecules dissociated per cell
1	fresh cells	anti-IgG	anti-SRBC	2,200
2	fresh cells	PAP	anti-SRBC	2,000
3	fresh cells	DAB	anti-SRBC	cells agglutinated *
4	cells reacted with anti-SRBC	PAP	anti-IgG	0
5	cells reacted with anti-SRBC	DAB	anti-IgG	200
6	cells reacted with anti-SRBC and anti-IgG	DAB	PAP	0

Sheep erythrocytes (SRBC) were reacted with rabbit serum anti-SRBC at a concentration known to bind one million sites per cell [Fig. 7-1(a)] and stained by the unlabeled antibody enzyme method. These cells are called "treated cells." To examine the dissociation of anti-SRBC, an equal number of fresh cells ("test cells") were added to the immunocytochemical staining reagents prior to admixture with the treated cells, and the number of deposits transferred to the fresh cells was counted upon completion of the staining procedure. For measurement of dissociation of anti-IgG from treated cells, test cells reacted with anti-SRBC (10^6 sites per cell) were added to the immunocytochemical reagents. Finally, to test dissociation of peroxidase-antiperoxidase complex (PAP) from treated cells, test cells reacted with anti-SRBC (1 million molecules per cell) and anti-IgG were added to the diaminobenzidine-hydrogen peroxide mixture before completing the staining sequence. SRBC, sheep erythrocytes, DAB, 0.05% diaminobenzidine and 0.01% hydrogen peroxide in 0.05 M Tris buffer, pH 7.6. From the work of Ludwig Sternberger.

* The test cells were agglutinated, and measurement of transference of anti-SRBC was restricted to the outer surface of the agglutinate. Since in individual, agglutinated cells only part of the surface was exposed, the number of deposits recorded had to be integrated to total cell circumference. This led to an approximate value of 1,800 deposits per cell.

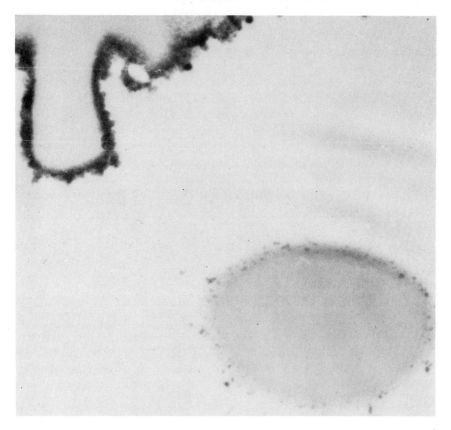

Fig. 7-3 The heavily stained cell membrane is a sheep erythrocyte (SRBC) that has bound 10^6 anti-SRBC molecules and has been further treated by the unlabeled antibody method. An equal number of fresh SRBC was added to the sheep serum antirabbit IgG prior to admixture with the treated cells. The cell at the right lower corner is one of these added cells. This cell has accepted on the average 2,000 molecules of anti-SRBC dissociated from the treated cells and stained by the unlabeled antibody enzyme method. X32,000. From the work of D. M. Hinton, J. P. Petrali, H. M. Meyer, and L. A. Sternberger.

and 7-4). The total loss of anti-SRBC during the entire staining procedure amounts to about 0.6% which is negligible compared to the over-all error in molecular immunocytochemistry.

Interestingly, no anti-IgG (Table 7-1, line 4) or only an insignificant number (line 5 and Fig. 7-5) is dissociated from the cell. The sheep serum anti-IgG is used in excess such as is available only in hyperimmune sera (the 1:10 dilution of the anti-IgG used in Table 7-1 contains 0.6 mg antibody per ml). The binding avidity of antibodies in hyperimmune sera is particularly strong, and by using the serum in excess, those antibodies of

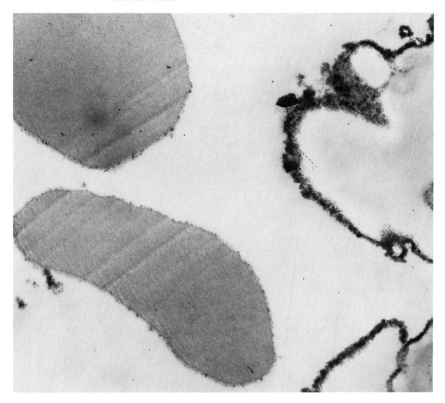

Fig. 7-4 Here the protocol resembled that of Fig. 7-4 except that the fresh cells were admixed to the PAP prior to addition to the treated cells. Heavy deposits are seen on the two treated cells (right), while the added fresh cells (left) have accepted an average of 2,000 anti-SRBC molecules that have dissociated from the treated cells after reaction with anti-IgG. X18,000. From the work of D. M. Hinton, J. P. Petrali, H. M. Meyer, and L. A. Sternberger.

highest avidities in the serum pool attach to the cells preferentially. This is reflected by low dissociation of the antibody during washing.

No PAP dissociates during incubation in diaminobenzidine and hydrogen peroxide (Table 7-1, line 6 and Fig. 7-6). This again is explained by the high avidity of the bound anti-IgG for the IgG in PAP (in each antibody molecule both antigen binding sites are identical and, hence, have equal avidities).

Some loss of peroxidase undoubtedly occurs from PAP during incubation in diaminobenzidine and hydrogen peroxide. However, this loss is small, because the circularity of PAP requires simultaneous release of peroxidase from two binding sites (the dissociation constant for PAP is 10^{-8}).

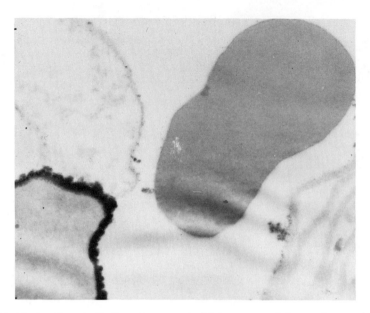

Fig. 7-5 The heavily stained cell membrane on the left lower corner is from a sheep erythrocyte (SRBC) that has bound 10^6 anti-SRBC molecules and has been treated by the unlabeled antibody enzyme method. An equal number of SRBC that have also bound 10^6 anti-SRBC molecules per cell but have not been reacted with anti-IgG was added to the DAB used for staining the treated cells. The cell in the center and the ghost on the upper left and lower right represent these added cells. Deposits on these added cells indicate dissociation of anti-IgG from the heavily stained cells during incubation with DAB. About 200 molecules of anti-IgG have been dissociated per cell. X20,800. From the work of D. M. Hinton, J. P. Petrali, H. M. Meyer, and L. A. Sternberger.

During washing after the diaminobenzidine and hydrogen peroxide step in the unlabeled antibody enzyme method, excess of polymerization reaction product is released from the cell suspension. Incomplete washing is responsible for loose reaction product occasionally seen in suspension (Fig. 7-6). This material does not reattach to tissue nonspecifically.

QUANTITATIVE IMMUNOCYTOCHEMISTRY

We have seen that in "molecular immunocytochemistry" enumeration of cellular antigens is only possible if they are well separated on a structure. Enumeration is precluded when antigen is closely packed, such as in secretion granules. In this case, however, antigen can be expressed in terms of concentration by optical density recordings of the granules on a photographic film. The procedure is restricted to post-embedding staining, in which experimental and control sections are prepared serially from the same block. In order to eliminate variation from section thickness and exposure time, densities are normalized by reference to organelles known to be free of the measured antigen. For instance, the density of cortico-

180

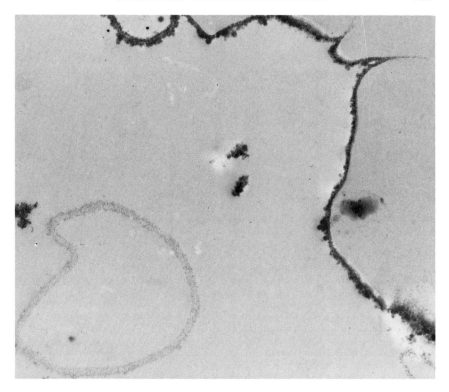

Fig. 7-6 The heavily stained membranes in the upper and right fields represent sheep erythrocytes (SRBC) that have bound 10^6 molecules anti-SRBC per cell and have been stained by the unlabeled antibody enzyme method. An equal number of SRBC that have bound 10^6 anti-SRBC molecules per cell and have been reacted anti-IgG, but not with PAP, was added to the diaminobenzidine and hydrogen peroxide prior to completion of the staining procedure. The cell at the left lower corner represents one of these added cells. It is free of attached deposits, showing that no PAP dissociated from the stained cells during incubation with diaminobenzidine and hydrogen peroxide. X20,000. From the work of D. M. Hinton, J. P. Petrali, H. M. Meyer, and L. A. Sternberger.

tropin secretion granules in the pituitary can be expressed in normalized form by reference to that of nuclear chromatin as follows:

$$\frac{[\text{density of secretion granules}] - [\text{density of nuclear chromatin}]}{[\text{density of nuclear chromatin}]}$$

In practice granules have been considered stained when the normalized density of an average of 100 to 600 granules differed from that in control sections at a significance of $P < .0001$. Similar significance requirements have been used to evaluate differences of dilutions of antisera and other staining reagents and variations in staining procedures. The details of the

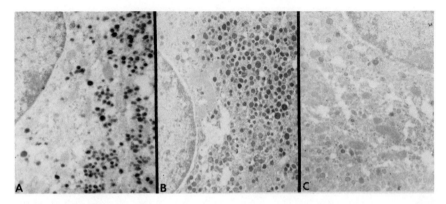

Fig. 7-7 These Araldite sections of glutaraldehyde-fixed rat pituitary intermediate lobe have been stained by the unlabeled antibody enzyme method using anti-[17-39] corticotropin as primary antiserum. The undiluted antiserum bound less than five nonagram of [17-39] corticotropin by radioimmunoassay. Micrograph A is the immunocytochemical localization after application of a 1:10,000 dilution of anti-[17-39] corticotropin followed by sheep antirabbit-IgG and PAP, diluted 1:50 to contain 0.066 μg antiperoxidase, and 0.024 μg peroxidase/ml. The normalized optical density of 596 granules was 0.294. In micrograph B, a 1:10,000 dilution of anti-[17-39] corticotropin was followed by sheep antirabbit-IgG, purified antiperoxidase and then by peroxidase. The antiperoxidase was diluted 1:5 to contain 0.066 μg antiperoxidase/ml. The normalized optical density of 612 secretion granules was 0.157. In micrograph C, a 1:10,000 dilution of anti-[17-39] corticotropin was followed by sheep antirabbit-IgG, rabbit antiserum to peroxidase and then by peroxidase. The antiserum was diluted 1:24 to contain 0.066 μg antiperoxidase/ml. The normalized optical density of 215 secretion granules was 0.019. The curves constructed for each of the three staining sequences by plotting densities against dilution of anti-[17-93] corticotropin showed that the unlabeled antibody enzyme method with PAP is 4 times more sensitive than with purified antiperoxidase and peroxidase, and 20 times more sensitive than with antiserum to peroxidase and peroxidase. From the laboratories of Ludwig Sternberger and Gwen Moriarty.

post-embedding staining protocol on page 158 were decided upon by these considerations.

Quantitative immunocytochemistry has shown that in the unlabeled antibody method the use of PAP is 4 times more sensitive than equal concentrations of specific antiperoxidase in a purified antiperoxidase preparation (85% pure) followed by peroxidase, and 20 times more sensitive than such concentrations of specific antiperoxidase in antiserum to peroxidase followed by peroxidase (Fig. 7-7). In the antiserum to peroxidase, 20% of total immunoglobulin was antiperoxidase. Therefore, we would expect antiserum and peroxidase to be $\frac{1}{5}$, and purified antibody and peroxidase to be 85/100 as sensitive as PAP. The increase of sensitivity differences between PAP and purified antiperoxidase beyond those expected is explained by avidity considerations (pages 2 and 176). During the reaction of anti-IgG with antiperoxidase, no selection is made between antibodies of high and low avidity for peroxidase. In the washing that follows application of peroxidase, enzyme is lost from antibodies of low avidity. When PAP is used instead of antiperoxidase and peroxidase, losses are minimal because the circularity of the complex provides for low dissociability of peroxidase.

The findings explain the failure of M. C. Willingham, S. S. Spicer, and C D. Graber to find enzyme-reaction product on lymphocytes stained for surface antigens by the unlabeled antibody enzyme method with the use of purified antiperoxidase followed by peroxidase and the usual washing procedure. Only when the cells were embedded in agar, after application of peroxidase and before incubation in diaminobenzidine and hydrogen peroxidase, did the surface become stained. Apparently, mechanical immobilization was necessary to maintain dissociated peroxidase in position. Unfortunately, embedding in agar may have interfered with removal by washing of excess of enzyme-reaction product. Instead, the product may have spread, during enzyme action, along the interspaces between cell and agar and may have resulted, for this reason alone, in a continuous distribution of deposits along the cell membrane. Thus, the data cannot be used to decide the controversy over patchy or continuous distribution of antigens on lymphocytes (page 106).

The loss of peroxidase from antiperoxidase, when applied separately, and the retention of peroxidase in PAP, where each enzyme molecule is held by two bonds, is reminiscent of the loss of ferritin from single, purified hybrid antibody molecules and its retention when simultaneously bound to several purified hybrid antibodies (page 98).

Comparison of the unlabeled antibody method using PAP and sequential application of antiperoxidase and peroxidase provides formal proof that the ring-shaped molecules observed in post-embedding staining with PAP (Fig. 6-24) are, indeed, PAP molecules: the ring-shaped structures are not observed when antiperoxidase and peroxidase are applied in sequence.

The peroxidase reaction product diffuses along membranes after its liberation at the enzyme site. Diffusion artifacts, described by Alex Novikoff and his associates, may make interpretation ambiguous when areas are viewed at high resolution. Immunostaining at high resolution must be confirmed by the presence of the characteristic PAP molecules on a specific structure. Absence of PAP precludes accurate interpretation of sequentially used antiperoxidase and peroxidase.

To obtain reproducible results in an immunocytochemical method, it is necessary that all reagents, except the primary antiserum, are used in excess. Quantitative immunocytochemistry has confirmed that a dilution of PAP containing 0.066 mg antiperoxidase/ml is excess for post-embedding staining. Staining intensity does not decrease markedly until less than 0.014 mg of PAP/ml are employed. However, 0.066 mg of specific antiperoxidase followed by peroxidase do not provide an excess of reagents. Decrease of the concentration of antiperoxidase below 0.066 mg greatly decreases staining intensity.

Gwen Moriarty and her associates used quantitative immunocytochemistry to determine the sensitivity of the unlabeled antibody PAP method as compared to radioimmunoassay. With anti-[17-39]corticotropin as primary antiserum, the sensitivity of immunocytochemistry exceeded that of radioimmunoassay 1,000-fold. The difference in sensitivity is presumably due to two factors: first, the unlabeled antibody enzyme method can detect single molecules, while radioimmunoassay only detects those molecules that decompose during the counting time. Second, anti-[17-39]corticotropin combines only with a small region of the whole corticotropin molecule. Therefore, no corticotropin can be bound to more than one antibody during radioimmunoassay, and dissociation occurs readily. Dissociation of antigen reduces the efficiency of the radioimmunoassay. In immunocytochemical assay, on the other hand, antigen is immobilized in the section. The primary antibody can bind two adjacent antigen molecules. Impairment of efficiency could occur, if the antibody dissociates. Since it is bound by two sites, its loss occurs only if both sites dissociate simultaneously.

When antiserum to whole corticotropin is used, immunocytochemistry is also more sensitive than radioimmunoassay, though to a lesser extent than with anti-[17-39]corticotropin. Antiserum to whole corticotropin, presumably, contains antibodies to N-terminal, as well as C-terminal portions of corticotropin. Therefore, antigen can undergo multiple binding with bivalent antibodies, thus, producing a polymeric lattice, or chain, and reducing greatly the chance of dissociation of antigen. The sensitivity of radioimmunoassay is, thereby, increased though not sufficiently to approach that of immunocytochemistry.

REFERENCES

Hinton, D. M., Petrali, J. P., Meyer, H. G., and Sternberger, L. A. The unlabeled antibody enzyme method of immunohistochemistry. Molecular immunocytochemistry of antibodies on the erythrocyte surface. *J. Histochem. Cytochem.*, 21:969, 1973.

Moriarty, G. C., Moriarty, C. M., and Sternberger, L. A. Ultrastructural immunocytochemistry by unlabeled antibodies and the peroxidase-antiperoxidase complex (PAP). A technique more sensitive than radioimmunoassay. *J. Histochem. Cytochem.*, 21:825, 1973.

Novikoff, A. B., Novikoff, P. M., Quintana, N., and Davis, C. Diffusion artifacts in 3,3'-diaminobenzidine cytochemistry. *J. Histochem. Cytochem.*, 20:745, 1972.

Willingham, M. C., Spicer, S. S., and Graber, C. D. Immunocytologic labeling of calf and human lymphocyte surface antigens. *Lab. Invest.*, 25:211, 1971.

Chapter 8

The Immune Response

Individuality has made its fossil imprint only in recent life on earth. In Precambrian times of monocellular existence, each cell among large populations of cells had a similar genetic endowment and was about equally susceptible to damaging influence: a rise in temperature of the environment could eliminate the whole species. Save for mutation, survival of the species only occurred if the damaging influence was geographically more limited than the species.

With the advent of the *fertility factor,* at least a few cells attained the chance opportunity to acquire chromosomal material from another cell through a sexual process and to assume, thereby, new genetic characteristics. Nonmutationally acquired characteristics have become wholly or in part transmissible from cell to cell, and variation among cells has increased. The greater the variation among cells the greater the chance for a few to possess stamina for survival under damaging influences.

Sexuality and reproduction are unlinked phenomena in unicellular organisms. Cell division still is *clonal;* each daughter cell still is the exact nonindividualistic replica of the mother cell.

However, during the last half billion years organisms appeared on earth that exhibited increasing preference to reproduce as a result of sexual union. In contrast to unicellular organisms in which the frequency of sexual union is rare relative to reproduction, the reverse becomes true, as we move along in vertebrate evolution. Obligatory sexuality insures that no offspring, unless they are identical twins, possess equal genetic endowment. No animal, and not even man, is born equal. Chance endowment makes everyone an individual.

As we have been vertebrate individuals for generations, the complexity of individual differentiation is so great that it is not surprising that no form of psychologic testing or theory permits dissection of individuality into definable components. However, there is one system that permits molecular separation of at least one form of individuality. The *immune response* is an individualistic endowment. Everyone of us is given a very large number of *preformed receptors* among which each has individual specificities. In an immune response antibodies are not formed around a templet. They are reproduced from preexisting endowment. Immunization is reproduction of a predestined, hypervariable region sequence (page 2) as a result of the interaction of an antigenic determinant with a *selected cell*. The ability to evoke antibodies against a particular external, damaging influence, such as measles virus, is a genetic characteristic that not only may help most of us to survive measles but also may have selected survival of our ancestors to beget us in an environment in which measles is occasionally epidemic.

Antibodies, and thus variable region individuality, have made their evolutionary appearance only in vertebrates, long after the advent of sexuality and individuality. It follows that antibodies are not the only mechanism of defense against disease. Phagocytosis, the uptake of foreign particles by destructive cells, exists as a nonspecific response in invertebrates and, indeed, persists in vertebrates. In phagocytosis it is necessary for the damaging substance to interact directly with the phagocytic cell (leukocytes and monocytes in vertebrates and their analogues in invertebrates). This response is sufficiently efficient to insure survival among many species, such as among insects. It is insufficient for survival of man on infection with a virus specific for certain tissues, as for instance common cold specifically infecting mucous membrances of the upper respiratory tract. The virus does not directly interact with the phagocytic cell. Instead, tissue would first be destroyed, and only the destroyed tissue could be scavenged nonspecifically by the phagocytic cell. The appearance of specific, individual immunity in vertebrates has introduced a mechanism of defense against noxious stimuli, even when they are specific for selective tissues and do not interact directly with the phagocytic cells. However, just as embryonic development of the human kidney has to recapitulate the development of the kidney of fish, so does the specific immune response to a certain antigen encompass features of undifferentiated, nonspecific, nonindividualistic responses, such as clonal cell division. Thus, the stimulus for production of antibodies depends on two essential, but unrelated phenomena: that is, the recently acquired antigenic recognition and the phylogenetically older, irritant-evoked cell replication. Also, it is not surprising that individual antigen recognition is a property of selected cells among a population of cells belonging to the same group of cells that are responsible for phagocytosis in species lacking an immune response. These cells are the lmphocytes, which along with other white blood cells, are unique among the nongonadal cells of animals as free-floating in body fluids and being able to replicate with great rapidity under a variety of stimuli.

An immune response to a specific antigen when it leads to secretion of antibodies is initiated upon binding of antigenic determinants of an antigen by specific recognizing units on few, selected lymphocytes. The cells are transformed to clonally dividing cells in whose progeny newly replicated DNA codes towards assembly of specific antibody. In many immune responses helper cells that also possess specific antigenic determinants interact with the antibody-producing cells to promote the immune response. Macrophages also participate in some responses by modifying certain types of antigens. A *secondary response* to an antigen differs from a *primary response* by accelerated and magnified antibody production and is mediated by the presence of a greater number of specific antigen-recognizing cells and, also perhaps, by the presence of *educated* (antigen-stimulated) helper cells. Not each immune response leads to antibody secretion or cellular immunity. Instead, *tolerance,* a state of active refractoriness to antigen, may be induced, apparently by mediation through the helper cells.

Immunocytochemistry is important in describing initial events on the cell surface during selection of the receptor by antigen and during induction of cellular replication. Immunocytochemistry again becomes important in describing the final events of assembly of newly synthesized antibody.

In the restricted sense immunocytochemistry involves the detection of cellular antigens by the use of antibodies. In a broader sense immunocytochemistry includes the detection of antibodies. For this application special immunocytochemical methods that use antibodies as reagents are not necessary. Thus, antibodies to ferritin can be detected directly by a reaction with ferritin, antibodies to an enzyme by reaction with the enzyme and cytochemically visualizable substrate. Antibodies to other antgiens such as serum albumin can be detected with ferritin or enzyme-conjugated antigen. Alternatively, tritiated antigen can be used and the antigen-antibody reaction developed by application of the section to a photosensitive emulsion (such as Ilford L4), thus, using autoradiography in an immunocytochemical application. In immunofluorescence fluorescein-labeled antigen can be used if one is careful to limit the extent of labeling to about one molecule of fluorescein isothiocyanate per 100,000 daltons. This limitation makes labeling of antigen insensitive. A more sensitive procedure involves application of unlabeled antigen followed by fluorescein-labeled specific immunoglobulin.

Antigen Recognition

If a population of lymphocytes, such as obtained from normal mouse spleen or lymph nodes, is exposed to a specific antigen, such as bovine serum albumin, about 1 in 1,000 cells are found to bind antigen specifically. The cells so selected possess a *specific receptor* for bovine serum albumin. Binding is detected by immunocytochemical methods, such as immunofluorescence, or immunoferritin, or by autoradiography with ^{125}I-labeled antigen. If sheep erythrocytes (SRBC) are used as antigen, binding can be detected by formation of *rosettes* of SRBC around the few selected lymphocytes that bear SRBC-recognizing units on their surfaces. Cells with receptors to flagellin can be detected by binding and immobilization of specific flagellate bacteria and counted by formation of bacterial colonies upon plating on semisolid media. The proportion of cells revealing specific receptor varies with the sensitivity of the method of detection. Thus, A. Miller and co-workers show that when β-galactosidase or horseradish peroxidase is used as antigen and binding assayed cytochemically by specific chromogenic substrate, enzyme action provides a cytochemical amplifier, and the number of specifically marked normal lymphocytes increases to as many as 40 per 1,000 from the usual 1 per 1,000.

The specific binding of antigen upon contact with a few selected lymphocytes is *necessary* for initiation of the immune response. Elimination of specific receptor cells from a population of lymphocytes abolishes the immune response. The antibody-forming capacity of the cell population to a specific antigen can be deleted by passing the cells through a column of glass beads coated with the specific antigen. Also, radioactive antigen of high specific activity results in destruction of the specific receptor-bearing cells, while leaving the remaining cells unaffected: upon transfer of the cells to irradiated recipient animals, injection of unlabeled specific antigen fails to result in antibody formation, while unrelated antigen results in a normal response (the recipient animals are irradiated in this commonly used assay of antibody-producing cells *in vivo* in order to eliminate the host's own lymphoid cells, to permit a rapid replication of transferred cells, and to prevent graft rejection of the injected cells). The binding of a *hapten,* such as dinitrophenol (DNP), by receptor is less strong than the binding of moderately or heavily DNP-conjugated proteins (*hapten-carrier*), because the latter combines with multiple sites on the cell (binding avidity increases exponentially with the number of binding sites). Thus, pretreatment with *low concentrations* of DNP inhibits neither the binding of DNP-protein nor the immune response to the hapten. However, when DNP is converted to a compound that reacts covalently with protein [such as α-N-bromacetyl-ϵ-N-(2,4-dinitrophenyl) lysine], the hapten becomes an *affinity label* that reacts irreversibly with the receptor with a high degree of specificity. Subsequent exposure to DNP-protein fails to result in an anti-DNP response.

Reaction of an antigen with a specific lymphocyte receptor, although a necessary condition for initiation of an immune response, is not a sufficient condition. Other factors, independent of the specificity of recognition, determine whether and to what extent cellular transformation and replication will occur, and what class of antibody, if any, will be produced.

The specificity of the receptor is the only known mechanism of selection of the specificity of the antibody produced. However, if as many as 4% of lymphocytes specifically recognize a single antigen, such as β-galactosidase, and if these cells recognize only this antigen to the exclusion of other antigens, there could not be formed more than 25 different noncross-reacting antibodies to protein. In fact, however, thousands of different noncross-reacting antibody specificities and millions of different, though cross-reacting hypervariable region sequences can be formed by an individual. It follows that subsequent to the first encounter with antigen there must be some selection of the most specific receptor.

Binding of β-galactosidase can be observed cytochemically by using 5-bromo-4-chloro-3-indol-β,D-galactoside as substrate to yield in oxygen an insoluble indigo blue reaction product deposited in the vicinity of the receptor-bearing cell. Binding of peroxidase can be evaluated on cell populations treated with hydrazine to destroy intrinsic peroxidase activity. Hydrogen peroxide substrate with 3-amino-9-ethyl carbazol as hydrogen donor yields a red indamine reaction product with peroxidase. The frequency of cells revealing both blue and red deposits and, therefore, accepting both enzymes approximates the product of frequencies of cells staining only blue for β-galactosidase and only red for peroxidase. If fluorescein-di-β-galactoside is used as substrate for β-galactosidase, sensitive fluorescence assay of the free fluorescein reaction product provides measurement of the product of a single enzyme molecule. When enzyme-treated, washed lymphocytes are placed into microdroplets along with the substrate, release of reaction product from a single cell and the number of specific enzyme receptors per cell can be measured. This number exhibits great variation from cell to cell, ranging from 30,000 to 1,000,000. Even the maximum number is smaller than that required to saturate the cell surface with protein (page 173) and allows for the presence of other factors besides receptors on the cell surface. The observed variation in number of receptor molecules can be interpreted by assuming a variable heterogeneity of receptors on cells: the cells with one million receptors are more homogenous and bear receptors of only one or few specificities. The cells with 30,000 receptors are more heterogenous and bear receptors of many different specificities, most of which are directed towards antigens other than that examined. Alternatively, the receptor population on each cell may be homogenous, but there may be affinity variations of receptor from one cell to another. Thus, cells that bind 1,000,000 galactosidase molecules are high affinity binders for this antigen, while cells that bind 30,000 galactosidase molecules are probably highly avid for another antigen and react with galactosidase with the low avidity characteristic of a cross-reaction.

During the course of immunization, the specificity of secreted antibodies continually changes towards increasing avidity and decreasing heterogeneity. The smaller the amount of antigen the greater the selection towards increased avidity, although total antibody protein evoked is diminished. The avidity of receptor on antigen-recognizing cells also increases during the course of immunization. J. Davie and W. Paul have measured avidity of guinea pig perpiheral and lymph node lymphocytes for DNP by the concentrations of DNP-lysine that inhibit binding of radioiodinated DNP-guinea pig albumin, containing 16 DNP groups per molecule of protein. DNP-lysine binds monovalently with the DNP receptor, but the DNP serum albumin binds polyvalently and, hence, practically irreversibly. Thus, the inhibitory concentration of DNP-lysine becomes essentially inversely proportional to the avidity of the receptor. Following a single injection of DNP-guinea pig serum albumin, there is a rapid increase in receptor-bearing cells to about 10-fold their initial number on the 8th day and 50-fold on the 20th day. The number of receptor sites per cell also increases. After the 20th day a plateau level of newly formed receptor cells is maintained. These newly formed receptor cells are called *memory cells*. They offer a larger number of receptors to a repeat (secondary) injection of antigen and provide for a boosted reinitiation of the immune response. The average binding avidity of receptor before a primary injection and up to the 6th day is about 10^{-3}. After the 6th day there is a rapid increase in binding avidity, reaching 3×10^{-4} on the 7th day, 10^{-5} on the 18th day, 10^{-7} on the 22nd day, and 10^{-9} on the 30th day.

The increase in avidity of the receptor is paralleled by an increase in avidity of the antibody that is produced by the progeny of the receptor-bearing cell. This is assayed by injecting receptor-bearing cells into irradiated, isogeneic guinea pigs followed one day later by dinitrophenyl (DNP)-hemocyanine and four days later by normal guinea pig bone marrow cells to sustain the irradiated guinea pigs. The number of antibody producing cells in the cell suspension obtained from the guinea pigs on the sixth day is measured by plating a mixture of cells and 2,4,6-trinitrobenzene sulfonic acid-conjugated sheep erythrocytes on agar in the presence of complement. The number of IgM anti-DNP producing cells corresponds to the number of hemolytic plaques. For assay of the number of IgG anti-DNP producing cells, rabbit serum anti-guinea pig IgG is added in order to facilitate efficient fixation of complement (anti-IgG aggregating with the guinea pig IgG, page 11). Addition of increasing concentrations of

DNP lysine to the culture medium progressively inhibits plaque formation. At low concentrations of DNP-lysine, only high avidity antibodies are prevented from producing hemolysis. At any concentration of DNP-lysine, antibodies of avidities higher than that given by this concentration will be inhibited. The number of hemolytic plaques that do form reflects, therefore, the cell fraction that produces antibodies of avidities lower than that given by the concentration of DNP-lysine. By varying the concentration of DNP-lysine, it is possible to determine which fraction of a cell population produces antibodies within a certain avidity range. On the sixth day after the primary antigen injection, the avidity range of antibody-secreting cells is broad. Although the average avidity is relatively low, there already exist a few cells producing high avidity antibodies. By the eighth day the number of antibody-producing cells has greatly increased. Cells producing high and low avidity antibodies participate in this proliferation. After the 15th day the number of antibody-producing cells decreases (in distinction to the number of receptor cells). However, the decrease is mainly accounted for by cells producing low avidity antibodies. The number of cells producing high avidity antibody stays fairly constant. Therefore, the average avidity of the antibodies produced increases. Cells producing high avidity antibodies replicate even late after an injection of antigen.

The existence of high avidity antibody-producing cells early in immunization suggests that the potential for high avidity antibodies preexists probably in the form of a high avidity receptor. In other words the high avidity receptor is not the result of mutation or cellular interaction during immunization. The heterogeneity of avidity of early antibodies can be explained by heterogeneity of receptor-bearing cells, each possessing a single type of receptor of equal avidity. An alternative explanation would attribute to each cell a variety of receptors of unequal avidities of which all but one are restricted in expression during immunization. Early in immunization antigen concentration is high, thus, permitting binding with high and low avidity receptors and resulting in replication of a heterogeneous population of receptor cells. Later as antigen concentration decreases only the high avidity receptors bind, and only cells stimulated by this binding will replicate. Low avidity receptors or low avidity receptor cells disappear, and the antibody produced becomes of increasingly higher avidity. As at this time only high avidity receptor-stimulated cells replicate, the total number of receptor-bearing cells does not increase late in the immune response.

Once antibody is secreted, beginning with the seventh day, antigen is eliminated rapidly. The persistence of selection of high avidity receptor cells (memory cells) in large numbers beyond the 15th day after a primary, and even more so after a secondary response, requires the persistence of small amounts of antigen. Although antigen as such does not persist during this phase of the immune response, antigen in specially processed forms (pages 205–208) may provide the necessary stimulus. It is difficult to ascribe the persistence of high avidity receptor cells to the persistence of small amounts of unmodified antigen because small, subclinical amounts of an infectious antigen are more frequently encountered by normal hosts than large, clinically effective amounts. If these small amounts of infectious antigens evoke high avidity antibodies, there should be a wide distribution of high avidity natural antibodies against most organisms in normal hosts. This would be accompanied by the presence of a preponderance of high avidity receptor cells in normal hosts, while in fact, prior to immunization the population of receptor cells is highly heterogeneous. Natural antibodies also are characterized by rather low avidities, as illustrated by the low avidity of the DNP-reactive immunoglobulin secreted by the mouse plasmacytoma MOPC-315 (page 14).

Perhaps it is possible to invoke the role of antibody rather than of antigen in selecting the increasing avidity of antibody produced in the course of immunization. In fact until antibody is secreted, that is until the seventh day, the average avidity of the receptor increases little. However, once anti-DNP is secreted antibody to its idiotypic determinants may form. The idiotypic antibodies could react specifically with the DNP-receptor lymphocytes and suppress the immune response by competition with DNP-guinea pig albumin. The binding strength of reaction of the receptor with antigen depends on the avidity of the receptor. However, the binding strength of reaction of idiotypic antibody with receptor depends on the avidity of the antibody. There is, therefore, no a priori reason for expecting the idiotypic antibody to bind more strongly with high avidity than with low avidity receptors. Hence, idiotypic antibodies can compete more effectively with the binding of antigen to lower avidity than to high avidity receptors. As a result, there will be a selective suppression of low avidity receptors. Idiotypic antibody is expected to come into play at approximately 12–14 days after a primary immunization (6–7 days for formation of anti-DNP and 6–7 days for formation of idiotypic antibody). Indeed, it is after the 12th day that low avidity antibody-forming cells decline in number. The invocation of idiotypic antibodies in the control of avidity would explain why a high avidity antibody response follows a low avidity response rather than occurring as an early event after injection with minimal subimmunogenic amounts of antigen.

Neonatally thymectomized animals or congenitally athymic, "nude" mice are deficient in cellular immunity (hypersensitivity and transplant rejection) and in humoral antibody responses to most antigens. However, the humoral response to some antigens such as lipopolysaccharides remains unaffected. This phenomenon differentiates two types of lymphocytes, namely *T cells,* originally derived from the *T*hymus, and *B cells* originally derived from the *B*ursa of Fabricius in birds and from the *B*one marrow in the case of mice. Both cells are morphologically identical. Both cells possess specific receptors for antigen. They can be distinguished cytochemically by antigenic determinants on their surfaces. For description of thymus, bursa, and bone marrow, see L. Weiss, *The Cells and Tissues of the Immune System,* Prentice-Hall, Inc., Englewood Cliffs, N. J., 1972.

T Cell Markers

T cells in mice bear θ-antigen, an allelic marker detectable, for instance, in C3H mice by fluorescein-labeled AKR mouse serum anti-C3H thymocytes. The antigen is absent from neonatally thymectomized or nude mice. Therefore, θ is a marker for T cells.

Cells bearing specific receptors for sheep erythrocytes can be detected by *rosette formation* (a rosette is a lymphocyte surrounded by attached erythrocytes). Reaction of antibody with an antigenic determinant on or near the specific receptor blocks rosette formation. Thymic lymphocytes contain a high proportion of θ-bearing lymphocytes, as evident by decrease in rosette formation after reaction with anti-θ serum. Comparison of the decrease in number of rosette-forming cells in thymic and peripheral lymphocytes as a result of reaction with antibodies against any receptor-associated antigen determines, therefore, whether the receptor is carried by T or B cells or both. Alternatively, the effect of antibodies on lymphocytes from normal mice and from B cell-selected (T cell-depleted) mice may be compared. Either "nude" mice can be used as depleted mice or depletion can be accomplished by thymectomy, and chronic thoracic duct canulution, or X radiation followed by reconstitution with anti-θ treated bone marrow.

The specific receptor on lymphocytes resembles a natural antibody not only because of its specificity, but also because it contains antigenic markers in common with humoral immunoglobulins. The resemblance to humoral immunoglobulins is greater for the B cell receptor than for the T cell receptor. However, even T cell rosette formation can be inhibited by antiserum against L-chain determinants. J. Marchalonis and co-workers report the isolation of a protein of about 200,000 molecular weight from human and murine neonatal thymic lymphocytes specifically labeled on their surfaces by enzymatic iodination (lack of enzyme penetration into the interior of the cell limits labeling to the surface). Isolation requires 9 M urea and 10% acetic acid indicating tight, but not covalent binding to the cells. The isolated protein precipitates with rabbit serum antimouse IgG. Following solution in 9 M urea, reduction and acetylation, labeled material is obtained that possesses electrophoretic mobility identical with L-chains, plus one or two more fractions that do not correspond in electrophoretic mobility to a known immunoglobulin chain.

T cell rosette formation can be inhibited by anti-μ. This inhibition is abolished by pretreatment of the anti-μ with IgM F(ab')$_2$ but not with IgM Fab. Therefore, the receptor presents antigenic determinants resembling the hinge region of the μ chain but not its more C-terminal portions. These data and the relative difficulty of extraction of receptor from the cell surface suggest that the T cell receptor, indeed, is an antibody that either is of a class different from humoral antibodies or alternatively, possesses an Fc portion that is deeply buried in the surface of the cell.

The nature of the immunity expressed by progeny of T cells resembles in several respects the nature of the receptor: T cells are responsible for cellular immunity that is mediated without influence of humoral antibodies. Tight attachment of antibody to the cell surface or complete burying in it may explain why this form of immunity is mediated only by direct cellular contact and not by circulating antibodies. Analysis of chromosomal markers shows that T cells are not precursors of cells forming humoral antibody.

B Cell Markers

In nonimmunized mice, rosette-forming B cells bear κ and μ *chain* determinants and occasionally α, γ_1, γ_{2a} and γ_{2b} determinants. The μ chain determinants on B cells, in contrast to those on T cells, react with anti-μ absorbed with IgM F(ab')$_2$. Thus, binding of antibodies specific to the C-terminal portion of heavy chains serves as a marker for B cells. Binding can be measured by immunofluorescence or other immunocytochemical means, by radioautography, or by inhibition of rosette formation.

S. Fröland, J. Natvig, and P. Berdal show by immunofluorescence that about 6% of peripheral human lymphocytes bear μ determinants and 5% γ determinants. Gamma$_2$ is the most common subclass; γ_1 and γ_3 are found occasionally. Alpha determinants are seen in 1% of cells.

In addition to receptors for specific antigen, B cells also possess receptors for Fc. Binding is weak. According to Basten and co-workers detection of receptors requires antigen-antibody complexes rather than antibody only. Apparently, binding is stabilized by the multiplicity of Fc

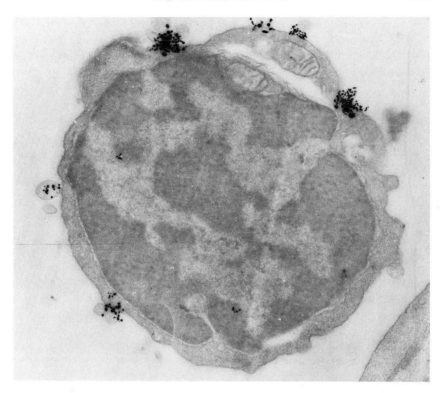

Fig. 8-1 Thoracic duct lymphocyte from an adult, thymectomized, irradiated CBA mouse protected with CBA bone marrow. The cell has been exposed *in vitro* to antigen-antibody complex consisting of ^{125}I-labeled fowl immunoglobulin and mouse (CBA) anti-fowl immunoglobulin. Dense patches of label are seen in spots on the cell surface after 14 days of exposure to Kodak NTE emulsion. X22,000. From A. Basten, N. C. Warner, and T. Mandel, *J. Exper. Med.,* **135**:627, 1972.

groups that is provided in antigen-antibody complexes. With the use of ^{125}I-labeled antigen in the antigen-antibody complex, the site of attachment to the B cell can be visualized by radioautography (Fig. 8-1). Antigen-antibody complex, thus, becomes another marker for B cells.

Chromosomal markers show that antibody-secreting cells and plasma cells are derived from B cells. With the acquisition of the property of secretion of highly specific, monoclonal antibody (homogeneous within each cell), plasma cells have lost several of the characteristics of the undifferentiated B lymphocyte: their surfaces bear no receptors for antigen, no light or heavy chain markers, and no receptors for antigen-antibody complex (Fc).

The unstimulated B cell may produce several classes of heavy chains. Takahashi and his co-workers find that in cell lines derived from a patient with acute lymphocytic leukemia and from one apparently normal individual a significant number of cells reveal mixed fluorescence (page 42) when stained with fluorescein-conjugated anti-γ and tetramethylrhodamine-conjugated anti-α.

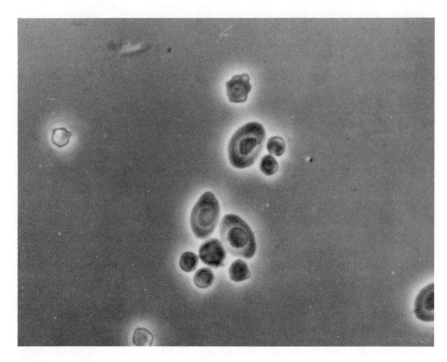

Fig. 8-2 A mixed rosette consisting of a central B lymphocyte surrounded by three ferritin-coated sheep erythrocytes and two ovalbumin-coated chicken erythrocytes. The rosette was formed by reaction with a mixture of hybrid antimouse-IgG/antiferritin and hybrid antimouse-IgF/anti-ovalbumin. Attachment of both the chicken and sheep erythrocytes to a single lymphocyte shows that the latter carries determinants for IgG as well as IgF. Formation of this rosette depended on the reaction of antibodies with antigen on the erythrocyte as well as on the lymphocyte. Such rosettes should not be confused with a rosette formed by "rosette-forming cells" in which a cellular receptor on the lymphocyte bears specificity for antigenic determinants on erythrocytes. From S. T. Lee, F. Paraskevas, and L. G. Israels, *J. Immunol.*, **107**:1583, 1971.

The majority of nonimmunized spleen cells of the mouse that carry γ-chains, possess determinants for both major mouse IgG subclasses. This is demonstrated by an immunocytoadherence test in the work of S. T. Lee, F. Paraskevas, and C. Israels in which the cells are reacted with two hybrid antibodies (Chapter 4). One is a hybrid antibody to mouse IgG and ferritin and the other a hybrid antibody to mouse IgF and ovalbumin. Sheep erythrocytes (nonnucleated) coated with ferritin and chicken erythrocytes (nucleated) coated with ovalbumin are used as indicator cells. Among 1,000 spleen cells about 300 carry γ determinants and are, therefore, B cells. Among these 300 cells, 200 form mixed agglutinates of nonnucleated and nucleated red cells (Fig. 8-2) upon reaction with both hybrid antibodies and with coated sheep and chicken erythrocytes. Therefore, $\frac{2}{3}$ of all reacting B cells carry determinants of both major mouse immunoglobulin classes.

Even four to seven days after a primary injection of sheep erythrocytes into mice, many rosette-forming cells (sheep erythrocyte receptor-bearing cells) may present more than one heavy chain class on their surfaces. However, 10 to 30 days after injection of antigen, only a single class is shown on any rosette-forming cells.

T. Kishimoto and K. Ishizaka find that even in a secondary response antigen receptor-bearing B cells of rabbits destined to differentiate into IgM-producing cells have both γ and μ determinants on their surfaces. This is demonstrated by suppression of IgM antibody production *in vitro* in the presence of either anti-γ or anti-μ.

While the presence of one or more class determinants on a single B cell is common, most, but not necessarily all, B cells possess even in heterozygous animals only one light and heavy chain allotype marker on their cell surface determinants.

CELL TRANSFORMATION AND DIFFERENTIATION

If an immune response ensues the cell whose specific receptor has reacted with antigen is induced to replicate. This process can be measured by incorporation of tritiated thymidine. The replicated cell still may bear antigen receptor on its surface, sometimes even in increasing numbers and, thus, is able to react with additional antigen. Such a second encounter with antigen induces even more cells to replicate and magnifies, thereby, the immune response. For this reason a secondary immune response is more rapid and leads to formation of larger amounts of antibodies than a primary immune response. However, along with replication, cells also may become more differentiated. They loose their surface antigen receptors and if they are B cells assume an enlarged cytoplasmic volume, containing at first the moderate amount of endoplasmic reticulum of the *blast cell* and eventually the profuse amount of endoplasmic reticulum of the differentiated *plasma cell*. Immunoglobulin specific to the immunizing antigen is found in the majority, but not in all blast and plasma cells (Figs. 8-3, 8-4, and 8-5). Although blast transformation is a prerequisite for eventual antibody secretion, both processes do partially overlap. J. Hay and his co-workers show that many cells that incorporate tritiated thymidine into

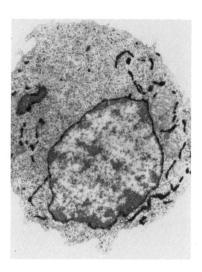

Fig. 8-3 This is a blast cell from the efferent lymph of a sheep after a secondary response to horseradish peroxidase. Cells have been fixed in 1.25% glutaraldehyde and exposed to 50 mg/ml of horseradish peroxidase for 30 minutes at room temperature, refixed in glutaraldehyde, stained with diaminobenzidine and hydrogen peroxide, fixed in osmium tetroxide and embedded in epon. Antiperoxidase is found in the perinuclear space, on cytoplasmic polyribosomes and in the endoplasmic reticulum. In these cells the Golgi region is usually not stained, even if the endoplasmic reticulum contains much antibody. There is no evidence of sequential appearance of antibody in any particular order. Thus, at times the perinuclear staining is absent. At other times the ribosomal staining is absent. X10,000. From J. B. Hay, M. J. Murphy, B. Morris, and M. C. Bessis, *Amer. J. Pathol.*, **66**:1, 1972.

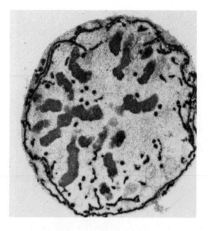

Fig. 8-4 A cell in mitosis that contains antiperoxidase. Blast transformation, cellular replication, and antibody secretion are not mutually exclusive. X10,000. From J. B. Hay, M. J. Murphy, B. Morris, and M. C. Bessis, *Amer. J. Pathol.*, **66**:1, 1972.

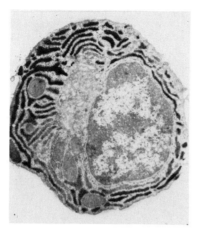

Fig. 8-5 A lymph node plasma cell 120 hours after a secondary challenge with horseradish peroxidase. Concentric channels of endoplasmic reticulum contain antibody. Such cells are never found in the efferent lymph. X10,000. From J. B. Hay, M. J. Murphy, B. Morris, and M. C. Bessis, Amer. J. Pathol., 66:1, 1972.

their nuclei as detected by autoradiography also contain specific antibody in their endoplasmic reticulum.

Although the early antigen-recognizing cell possesses determinants for various immunoglobulin classes, the transformed cell produces only one class. The loss of capability to produce different class determinants (class shift) proceeds independently of selection of immunoglobulin specificity. Guinea pigs immunized with highly substituted dinitrophenyl (DNP) bovine γ globulin produce IgG_1 and IgG_2 anti-DNP with fairly similar Fab regions. A. Eden, M. Lamm, and V. Nussenzweig have reduced, acetylated, and separated H- and L-chains from IgG_1 and IgG_2 anti-DNP preparations from individual animals. On readmixture they find that recombination of the H-chains with each other is class specific, while recombination of the H-chains with L-chains is not class specific. The data permit speculation that the antibody-producing cells are derived from B cells that bear a single group of antigen receptors (variable regions) but possess the capability of producing two classes of heavy chain constant regions. During differentiation, only the capability to produce one class is maintained in any one cell. Thus, antibodies apparently homogeneous in the variable but heterogeneous in the class-determining regions are circulating in the animal.

Antibodies secreted by an individual antibody-producing cell, be it a blast cell or a plasma cell, are always homogeneous. Antibodies of two specificities are never secreted by the same cell.

Even if immunization is carried out with two enzymes, such as peroxidase and phosphatase, so that antibodies can be revealed with high sensitivity after reaction with peroxidase and phosphatase and their respective cytochemical substrates to yield reaction products of contrasting color, S. Avrameas and his associates do not find cells that stain with both substrates.

Both T and B cells can undergo blast transformation, although only the latter differentiates into antibody-forming cells. T cells undergo processes of differentiation more related to cellular immunity. The initiation of blast transformation (thymidine incorporation) bears no relationship to specificity or avidity of the antigen receptor. It does bear a relation to the size of the antigen and the multiplicity of an antigenic determinant on the antigen. In fact blast transformation of lymphocytes is not unique to the immune response. Any stimulus that aggregates determinants on the cell surface is probably capable of initiating blast transformation. Thus,

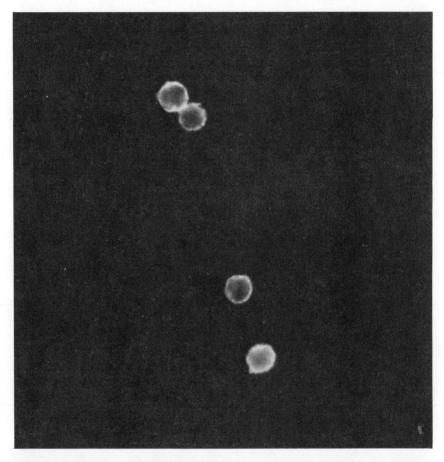

Fig. 8-6 Ring pattern of immunofluorescence of mouse-spleen cells, incubated in fluorescein-conjugated antimouse immunoglobulin at 0° C. X900. From R. B. Taylor, W. P. H. Duffus, M. C. Raff, and S. DePetris, *Nature, New Biology*, **233:**225, 1971.

T cells transform on stimulation with phytohemoagglutin. B cells can be transformed by anti-μ serum in the absence of specific antigen. We have already seen that reaction of a living cell with a bivalent antibody may cause a change in the distribution of a semiliquid antigen determinant on the cell, leading to aggregation and patch formation (page 103). On lymphocytes the phenomenon may have physiologic significance and may stimulate blast transformation. The aggregation requires an active cell capable of membrane flow and cell motility. When mouse spleen cells are stained in the cold with fluorescent rabbit antimouse immunoglobulin, R. Taylor, P. Duffus, M. Raff, and S. de Petris find a diffuse, ring-shaped pattern of fluorescence (Fig. 8-6). Upon staining at room temperature,

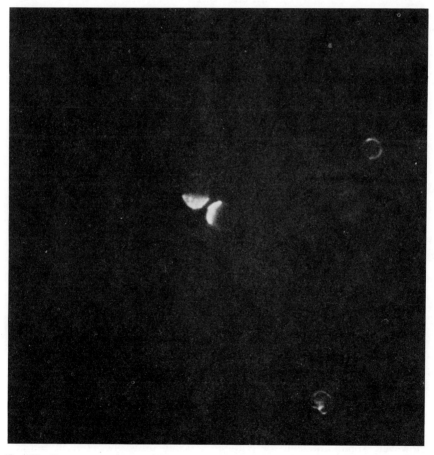

Fig. 8-7 Cap pattern of immunofluorescence of mouse-spleen cells incubated in fluorescein-conjugated antimouse immunoglobulin at room temperature. X1,000. From R. B. Taylor, W. P. H. Duffus, M. C. Raff, and S. DePetris, *Nature, New Biology,* **233:**225, 1971.

fluorescence aggregates as a cap on one pole of the cell (Fig. 8-7). With ferritin-labeled antibodies the cap is usually found at the uropod of the cell. Only ring fluorescence occurs upon staining with high concentrations of fluorescent antimouse immunoglobulin. Under these conditions only one antibody combining site reacts with the cell surface, and the other site remains free, thus, precluding aggregation of surface antigens. Cytocahalasin B that inhibits the contractile microfilament system responsible for cell movement also prevents cap formation, as do sodium azide or dinitrophenol. Cap formation is followed by rapid pinocytosis and, when ferritin-labeled antibodies are used, the ferritin is eventually found in the pinocytotic vesicles near the Golgi area.

HELPER FUNCTIONS

The ceaseless operation of essential functions throughout the life of an organism requires duplicated or alternate pathways, so that one pathway can take over when the other is damaged. In fundamental functions the alternate pathway is evoked easily. The complementary strand in the double helix fulfills an alternate function. When a base in one strand is damaged, the complementary strand determines the regeneration that follows excision. At times alternate pathways are invoked too slowly to sustain life, especially if the insult to the primary pathway is sudden and overwhelming. When acetylcholinesterase is poisoned, acetylcholine accumulates at the synaptic junction, and muscle paralysis ensues. However, within a few hours muscle contraction upon nerve stimulation returns through an adaptive pathway, despite the continued presence of excess acetylcholine and absence of functioning acetylcholinesterase. Unfortunately, this natural adaptation is too slow to sustain life of a poisoned individual.

Multiplicity forces itself upon us in nearly every immunologic phenomenon investigated. We have already seen that both light and heavy chains contribute to a single antibody combining site, and that the monomeric unit of antibody always contains two combining sites. Although an antigen receptor on a cell can react with a single antigenic determinant, such as a monovalent hapten, this interaction in itself will not initiate an immune response. Multiplicity of determinants, such as found in a polyvalent antigen, is necessary for cap formation and, thus, apparently for blast transformation. Antigens with regularly spaced, repetitive determinants, such as lipopolysaccharides, fulfill this requirement ideally; no wonder that they are excellent antigens that adhere strongly to cells and are capable of evoking as much as 35 mg of antibody per ml of serum. However, some antigenic determinants occur only once on an antigen molecule. Such antigens still are capable of invoking an immune response.

For instance, immunization with Fab will invoke, among others, antibodies against the L-chain, allotypic determinants that occur only on a single locus of the chain. To form antibodies against this determinant nature again invokes multiplicity. However, instead of using multiple bonding on a single cell the cooperation of a multiplicity of cells is involved. Both B and T lymphocytes are needed for the immune response against irregularly spaced determinants, such as determinants of native proteins or of haptens spaced irregularly on carrier proteins. Only B cells are needed for the immune response to lipopolysaccharides. Cooperation of B and T cells is not the only manner in which nature increases the antigenicity of a single determinant. The antigen itself can be modified, and its antigenicity multiplied by attachment to a repetitively structured backbone, such as RNA. In addition, during an immune response other helping and inhibiting factors are elaborated. Apparently, all these multiplicity functions express themselves via blast transformation as measured by incorporation of tritiated thymidine. They act independently of specificity itself. Although the avidity of antibody formed bears a direct relationship to the avidity of the cell receptor, incorporation of tritiated thymidine and the *amount* of antibody formed do not.

Antigens with repetitive subunit structure, such as polyvinylpyrolidon, lipopolysaccharides, pneumococcal polysaccharide, and bacterial endotoxin, that require only B cells do not even stimulate replication of T cells. *Brucella abortus,* ferritin, and polymerized flagellin, although not requiring T cells, do stimulate, according to J. Krüger and R. Gershon, thymidine incorporation in T cells. The subunit structure of these antigens is repetitive, but presumably not as regularly so as in lipopolysaccharides or polyvinylpyrolidon. Phytohemoagglutinin, on the other hand, stimulates T cells and leaves B cells unaffected. Most antigens require the cooperation of both cell types for humoral antibody formation. Hapten-carrier antigens offer the opportunity to dissect the contribution of each cell type.

While both B and T cells contain specific receptors, cellular cooperation is not dependent upon recognition of the same antigenic determinants. Indeed, the function of the carrier in permitting antihaptenic immunity depends upon recognition of the carrier and hapten by different cell types. It is possible to augment formation of anti-DNP after injection of DNP-hemocyanin by previous injection of hemocyanin alone. Thus, a secondary response to the carrier augments a primary response to the hapten.

The cooperation of T cells is essential for the production of antihaptenic antibody by B cells. An immune response is augmented if antigen is concentrated upon the receptor of the B cells. Thus, a secondary response in which the number of receptors per cell is high is stronger than a primary response in which the number of receptors per cell is lower. Immunogenicity of an aggregated antigen is stronger than that of a nonaggregated antigen and, as shown by G. Terres and his co-workers, the response to antigen-antibody complex (in antigen excess) is stronger than that to antigen alone. The effect of antigen-antibody complex is probably due to the Fc receptor characteristic of B cells. Mice immunized with a hapten-carrier, such as NIP-HGG (4-hydroxy-3-iodo-5-nitrophenyl-acetic acid azide conjugated into human immunoglobulin), are not appreciably stimulated by a secondary injection of NIP conjugated with a heterologous carrier such as fowl immunoglobulin. However, as shown by J. F. A. P. Miller and his associates, injection into irradiated hosts of a mixture of spleen cells of mice primed with NIP-HGG and washed B cells from other mice reacted with NIP-fowl immunoglobulin-antifowl immunoglobulin invokes a strong anti-NIP response. This response disappears when the T cells among the NIP-HGG-primed cells are eliminated by treatment with anti-θ serum and complement. Thus, the Fc receptor on B cells can enhance an immune response probably by increasing the binding strength of B cells and antigen, but it does not substitute for T cell-dependent responses. The response though of lesser magnitude can also be obtained with normal thoracic duct cells as a source of T cells. The enhanced response with spleen cells primed with NIP-HGG suggests that in this case B and T cells both cooperate after recognizing the haptenic determinant.

Recognition of the same determinant, however, is not necessary for the mechanism of cellular cooperation. A good system for the formation of a large number of antisheep erythrocyte (anti-SRBC)-secreting cells *in vitro* consists of a mixture of *educated* T cells and normal spleen cells. An increase in plaque-forming cells can be demonstrated with increase in the number of added T cells. Educated T cells are obtained from irradiated mice injected with syngeneic, thymic cells, and antigen (SRBC). The B cells are obtained from the spleens of thymus-deprived mice. Following culture of the cell mixture in the presence of sheep erythrocytes (SRBC), plaque-forming cells are assayed on a semisolid medium containing SRBC. Addition of the SRBC-educated T cells to the B cells increases the number of plaques formed by B cells. Philippa Hunter and her associates show that when the T cells are educated with donkey erythrocytes (DRBC), rather than with SRBC, their admixture with B cells fails to increase the number of plaques formed. Thus, a restimulation of the T cells in culture with specific "educating" antigen is required to augment production of anti-SRBC. If in addition the SRBC in culture are replaced by DRBC again, no increase in anti-SRBC forming plaques is observed. Although the educated T cells are restimulated with homologous antigen, plaque formation is inhibited because the B cells are not exposed to specific antigen.

However, DRBC-educated T cells do augment plaque formation of B cells on SRBC if both SRBC and DRBC are added to the culture medium. The findings show that T cells must undergo a specific immunologic response in order to exert helper function on B cells, but that the response does not necessarily have to be directed to the same antigen.

Similarly, as shown by A. Rubin and A. Coons, spleen cells of mice primed with tetanus toxoid release, upon culture in the presence of tetanus toxoid, a soluble factor that enhances the plaque formation of normal spleen cells cultured in the presence of SRBC. Again the release of the factor is specific, but its action is nonspecific: it augments the response of cells forming antibodies to an unrelated antigen. However, the timing of the effect appears to be critical. The enhancing factor is active on the second day of incubation of the plaque-forming cells with SRBC. It is not active when added on day 0. Apparently, the factor acts in the replication rather than the recognition phase of the immune response. The release of the factor from the sensitized cells is also time dependent. If this factor, indeed, is the substance needed for B and T cell cooperation, it requires appropriate timing of the B and T cell response to an antigen. Such timing may become assured if the B and T cell receptor-binding antigenic determinants are found on the same antigen molecule. Thus, a carrier may augment antihapten response, even though carrier and hapten are recognized by different cells.

R. Cone and A. Johnson show that polyadenylic-polyuridylic double helical complexes provide an *adjuvant* that greatly increases the response to many antigens. One of the pathways of mediation of the adjuvant effect is via proliferation of T cells. The adjuvant also affects macrophages (page 208) but has no effect on B cells.

Cell cooperation is not the only pathway through which an immune response can be augmented. Strong binding of antigen with the B cell is another, apparently, unrelated factor. Rough strains of pneumococci provide an excellent antigen apparently active only via B cells. H. McDonald, G. Odstrchel, and P. Maurer find that admixture of an otherwise poorly immunogenic haptenic polymer with rough strain pneumococci invokes an antihapten response of as much as 16 mg antibody per ml.

According to S. Sell and his co-workers, contact with cells must be prolonged to result in blast transformation. Antiimmunoglobulin allotype antibodies react with lymphoid cells and lead to blast transformation. Addition of excess of antigen (allotype-specific immunoglobulin) releases the antibodies competitively. If this addition is done within 36 hours after contact of cells with antibody, blast transformation is reverted. This confirms the need of strongly binding antigens for immunogenicity and explains why haptens that bind more reversibly are not immunogenic.

Among the lymphoid cells that infiltrate a lesion provoked by antigen, only some are antibody-producing cells containing antibody that can be detected by immunocytochemical means. Others may be cooperating cells. However, antigenic stimulation does not only result in blast transformation of specific receptor bearing cells. R. Levy and S. Rosenberg find that sensitized lymph node cells form new protein within four hours of incubation with specific antigen, that is, prior to cellular replication. The formation of this protein is associated with release of a mediator from the sensitized cells that recruits nonsensitized cells towards increased rate of protein synthesis.

Polymerization of a protein not only increases its specific binding with receptor lymphocytes and its antigenicity but also its nonspecific binding. Thus polymerized proteins become a source of nonspecificity in immunocytochemical methods (pages 84 and 126). Nonspecific binding on macrophages precedes nonspecific phagocytosis. D. Hirsh and his co-workers show that macrophage phagocytosis is not responsible for the enhanced antigenicity of aggregated trinitrophenyl (TNP)-hemocyanin. Indeed, macrophage phagocytosis diminishes the response by removing aggregated antigen from availability to specific receptor cells. However, macrophages do provide an alternate pathway for antigens that are not sufficiently aggregated to be strongly bound on receptor lymphocytes. Highly soluble (TNP)-hemocyanin is less antigenic than the polymerized form. Also, it is less efficiently phagocytosed by macrophages. However, antigen associated with macrophages obtained by washing the cell suspension invoked after interperitoneal injection of soluble TNP-hemocyanin is by far more immunogenic than soluble antigen alone. A unique ribonucleoprotein can be extracted from macrophages that binds antigenic fragments not larger than 3,600 daltons. This antigen RNA complex described by A. Gotlieb is highly antigenic. It provides an alternate pathway by which antigenic determinants on small molecules can evoke an immune response without need for polymerization or for possessing repetitive antigenic determinants.

Still another pathway towards induction of the immune response is mediated by an informational RNA. It differs from the RNA-protein antigen in its resistance to proteolysis. The informational RNA invokes antibody production by nonimmunized spleen cells. Clara Bell and S. Dray find that the majority of plaque-forming cells derived from such nonimmunized spleen cells produce light and heavy chain allotypes, belonging to the RNA donor rather than the cell donor. This provides evidence that not only the specific site but also part of the constant region of light and heavy chains are coded by informational RNA. S. Kurashige and S. Mitsuhashi have shown that informational RNA is capable of inducing

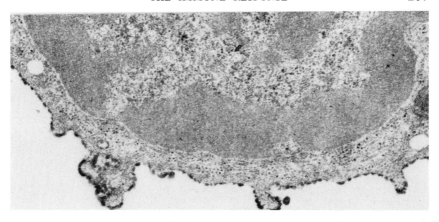

Fig. 8-8 A lymphocyte reacted with peroxidase-antiperoxidase complex (PAP) in the presence of complement reveals a regular and extensive distribution of the complement receptor on the cell surface. Each spot measures about 30 nm and probably represents a single PAP-complement complex. About 20% of lymphocytes obtained from mouse lymph nodes are capable of binding PAP. X35,000. In the absence of complement (not shown), only few spots are seen, and most of the cell surface is free of PAP. These spots appear as large clumps representing an aggregate of many PAP molecules. Apparently their binding is due to the Fc receptor on lymphocytes [page 194] (from the work of Li T. Chen and Leon Weiss). These observations suggest that binding by the Fc receptor is weaker than by the complement receptor. Apparently, PAP bound to a single Fc receptor is lost during washing in the processing of the cell, and only those PAP molecules are retained for observation that have bound more than one Fc receptor. In turn several PAP's could be bound by a single receptor-bearing molecule if each molecule possessed more than one receptor. The ensuing multiple binding could result in aggregation of the Fc receptors into clumps by movement on the cell surface (page 103). In the case of strong binding—such as apparently occurs with the complement receptor—a PAP molecule attached by a single bond is not washed off during processing of the cell and is retained for observation. No aggregation of cell surface receptor is expected upon such single site binding, thus, explaining the relatively uniform distribution of PAP on the complement receptor lymphocyte. Complement receptor can also be demonstrated by rosette formation of the B cell with sheep erythrocytes sensitized with anti-erythrocyte antibody and complement. As shown by L. T. Chen, A. Eden, V. Nussenzweig, and L. Weiss, the complement receptor lymphocyte can be dissociated from the erythrocytes in the rosette by Fab fragments of anti-C3 (monovalent), and the freed lymphocyte can be isolated. Occasionally this isolated lymphocyte still has attached to its surface small fragments of a sensitized erythrocyte.

memory functions on serial passage through isogeneic mice; that is, each recipient mouse undergoes a secondary response upon injection of a single dose of specific antigen. This function of the RNA is inhibited by administration of actinomycin D, showing that the informational RNA is replicated in the host after transfer. The size of immunogenic RNA and the effects of actinomycin suggest that informational RNA is not a messenger. Instead, the findings invoke the possibility that RNA may act as an episome that requires a "reverse transcriptase" (RNA-dependent DNA polymerase) for incorporation into the genome of the antibody-producing cell.

Polyadenylic-polyuridylic double helical complexes provide an adjuvant that enhances the uptake of ^{3}H-uridine into macrophages and the antigen-dependent stimulation of informational RNA. Both effects are again abolished by actinomycin D.

Another pathway for antigen may be provided by complement receptor lymphocytes. These are B cells that form rosettes with sheep erythrocytes sensitized by antibody and complement. The specific receptor on the lymphocyte reacts with C3 in distinction to the Fc receptor on B cells (Fig. 8-8). P. Dukor, C. Bianco, and V. Nussenzweig find that injected, sensitized, and complement-reacted erythrocytes adhere to lymphocytes in the follicular area, and the marginal zone of the spleen, and in the true cortex of the lymph nodes, sites of concentration of B cells. During immunization, lymphocytes form nodules as they concentrate around the processes of dendritic reticular cells. Antigen also binds on these processes. The adhesive function of C3, thus, may provide a mechanism for concentration of lymphocytes to follicular areas during the course of immunization. For a full treatment of cellular and tissue responses, see part III of L. Weiss, *The Cells and Tissues of the Immune System,* Prentice-Hall, Inc., Englewood Cliffs, N. J., 1972.

In *summary,* there appear to be multiple pathways by which an antigen may be accepted by immunocompetent cells in preparation for the production of humoral antibodies. Polymerized antigens may require solely the binding by specific receptor-bearing B cells. Most antigens also require specific binding by T cells and subsequent nonspecific cooperation between B and T cells. Antigens may be modified by attachment of relatively small molecular units to RNA. In addition, an informational RNA evoked by antigen may induce other cells to produce antibodies via a DNA-dependent mechanism. Instead of using specific antigen receptor, antigen may be bound to lymphocytes as antigen-antibody complex via the Fc receptor or as antigen-antibody-complement complex via the C3 receptor. Nonspecific substances induced early after antigenic stimulation amplify cell replication not only in the stimulated lymphocytes but also in surrounding cells. The selective theory of antibody production requires that immune responses in which antigen is modified via alternate pathways do involve at least at one point recognition by specific receptor units, such as provided by B or T cells.

IMMUNE TOLERANCE

The binding of an antigen on a receptor depends on avidity which in turn increases exponentially with the multiplicity of effective binding sites on an antigen molecule. It follows that with each antigen there is a limiting dose below which no immune response can be measured. Similarly, one can expect a limiting dose below which antigen may not be elaborated via alternate pathways. However, if antigen does become immunologically recognized the response is not necessarily *immunogenic* in that humoral antibody becomes produced or cellular immunity evoked. Instead, the response may be tolerogenic in that no immunity results. Tolerance is an active process. Injection of an *immunogen* after induction of tolerance by a *tolerogen* again fails to evoke immunity.

Immune tolerance is the fashionable response in embryonic life where immune response is thought to be immature. An antigen that is mainly an immunogen in adulthood may at the same dose level be primarily a tolerogen in immature animals. Tolerogenicity is favored over immunogenicity with increase of the dose of antigen and with the state of disaggregation of antigen. When a preparation of human immunoglobulin is centrifuged at high speed, the sediment consisting of aggregated immunoglobulin is an immunogen, while the supernatant is primarily a tolerogen, even to adult animals. Similarly, heat-aggregated human immunoglobulin becomes a good immunogen.

For responses to antigens that require both B and T cells, tolerance in either B or T cells prevents antibody formation. Irradiated mice reconstituted with thymus cells tolerant of human immunoglobulin and with normal spleen cells do not form antibodies after injection of aggregated human immunoglobulin. Irradiated mice reconstituted with bone marrow cells tolerant of human immunoglobulin and with normal thymus cells again fail to form antibodies after injection of aggregated human immunoglobulin. Tolerance is more rapidly induced in thymus cells than in bone marrow cells, and bone marrow cells, apparently, do not become tolerant in the absence of T cells. Therefore, it is believed that tolerance is a form of immune response characteristic to T cells, and that the T cells elaborate after reaction with a tolerogen, an effector that suppresses antibody formation by B cells. This sequence is similar to the elaboration by T cells after reaction with an immunogen of a factor that stimulates antibody formation by B cells. W. Droege finds that transferred, adult chicken thymus cells magnify the otherwise immature (weak or absent) antibody response of ten-day old chicks. The magnitude of the responses further increases if the transferred thymus cells are obtained from adult bursectomized (B cell-deficient) chickens, indicating that T cells, especially B cell-independent T cells subpopulations, have an immunogenetic effect. On the other hand, in adult chickens that possess a mature immune response expressed by antibody formation, injection of normal adult thymus cells suppresses the immune response. Interestingly, injection of thymus cells from adult, bursectomized chickens leaves the immune response substantially unaltered.

Apparently, a second subpopulation of T cells that is bursa-dependent exerts a tolerogenic effect.

We have seen that antibody in the form of antigen-antibody complexes (in antigen excess) may enhance an immune response (page 204). The effect is due to Fc receptors on B cells. M. Feldmann and E. Diener have shown that small amounts of antibody are able to confer tolerogenicity upon polymerized flagellin (a T cell-independent antigen). The effect is not due to Fc receptor cells, since $F(ab')_2$ is also effective. However, Fab' is ineffective. This suggests that bivalence of antibody is needed, and that antibody interspaced among antigenic determinants presents to the antigen receptor-bearing cells an arrangement especially suited for tolerogenicity.

REFERENCES

Abdou, N. I. Immunoglobulin (Ig) receptors of human peripheral leukocytes. II. Class restriction of Ig receptors. *J. Immunol.,* **107**:1637, 1971.

Avrameas, S., Taudou, B., and Ternyck, T. Specificity of antibodies synthesized by immunocytes as detected by immunoenzyme techniques. *Int. Arch. Allergy Appl. Immunol.,* **40**:161, 1971.

Blasten, A., Miller, J. F. A. P., Sprent, J., and Pye, J. A receptor for antibody on B lymphocytes. I. Method of detection and functional significances. *J. Exp. Med.,* **135**:610, 1972.

Basten, A., Warner, N. L., and Mandel, T. A receptor for antibody on lymphocytes. II. Immunochemical and electron microscopic characteristics. *J. Exp. Med.,* **135**:627, 1972.

Bell, C. and Dray, S. Conversion of nonimmune rabbit spleen cells by ribonucleic acid of lymphoid cells from an immunized rabbit to produce IgM and IgG antibody of foreign heavy-chain allotype. *J. Immunol.,* **107**:83, 1971.

Chen, L. T., Eden, A., Nussensweig, V., and Weiss, L. Electron microscopic study of the lymphocytes capable of binding antigen-antibody-complement complexes. *Cell Immunol.,* **4**:279, 1972.

Cline, M. J., Sprent, J., Warner, N. L., and Harris, A. W. Receptors for immunoglobulin on B lymphocytes and cells of cultured plasma cell tumor. *J. Immunol.,* **108**:1126, 1972.

Cone, R. E. and Johnson, A. G. Regulation of the immune system by synthetic polynucleotides. IV. Amplification of proliferation of thymus-influenced lymphocytes. *Cell. Immunol.,* **3**: 283, 1972.

Davie, J. M. and Paul, W. E. Receptors on immunocompetent cells. IV. Direct measurement of avidity of cell receptors and cooperative binding of multivalent ligands. *J. Exp. Med.,* 135:643, 1972.

Davie, J. M. and Paul, W. E. Receptors on immunocompetent cells. V. Cellular correlates of the "maturation" of the immune response. *J. Exp. Med.,* 135:661, 1972.

Davie, J. M., Paul, W. E., Mage, R. G., and Goldman, M. B. Membrane-associated immunoglobulin of rabbit peripheral blood lymphocytes: Allelic exclusion at the *b* locus. *Proc. Natl. Acad. Sci.,* U.S., 68:430, 1971.

Droege, W. Amplifying and suppressive effect of thymus cells. *Nature,* 234:549, 1971.

Dukor, P., Bianco, C., and Nussenzweig, V. Tissue localization of lymphocytes bearing a membrane receptor for antigen-antibody-complement complexes. *Proc. Natl. Acad. Sci.,* U.S., 67:991, 1970.

Eden, A., Lamm, M. E., and Nussenzweig, V. Complementarity of H and L chains from antihapten antibodies of different classes. *J. Immunol.,* 108:1605, 1972.

Feldmann, M. and Diener, E. Antibody-mediated suppression of immune response *in vitro.* IV. The effect of antibody fragment. *J. Immunol.,* 108:93, 1972.

Fröland, S., Natvig, J. B., and Berdal, P. Surface-bound immunoglobulin as a marker of B-lymphocytes in man. *Nature New Biol.,* 234:251, 1971.

Gallo, R. C. RNA-dependent DNA polymerase in viruses and cells: Views on the current state. *Blood,* 39:117, 1972.

Gershon, P. K., Cohen, P., Hencin, R., and Liebhaber, S. A. Suppressor T cells. *J. Immunol.,* 108:586, 1972.

Gery, I., Kruger, J., and Spiesel, S. F. Stimulation of B-lymphocytes by endotoxin. Reactions of thymus-deprived mice and karyotypic analysis of dividing cells in mice bearing T_6T_6 thymus grafts. *J. Immunol.,* 108:1088, 1972.

Gottlieb, A. A., Schwartz, R. H., and Waldman, S. R. Competition between L- and D-synthetic copolymers at the level of macrophage. *J. Immunol.,* 108:719, 1972.

Greaves, M. F., Torrigiani, G., and Roitt, I. M. Inhibition of human mixed lymphocyte reaction by antibodies to immunoglobulin. *Clin. Exp. Immunol.,* 9:313, 1971.

Hay, J. B., Murphy, M. J., Morris, B., and Bessis, M. C. Quantitative studies on the proliferation and differentiation of antibody-forming cells in lymph. *Am. J. Path.,* 66:1, 1972.

Hirsh, D. C., Amkrant, A. A., and Steward, J. P. Effect of carrier modification on the cellular and serologic responses of the rat to the TNP hapten. I. Dependence of the immunogenicity of the antigen upon processing by macrophages, as well as upon the distribution and retention of the antigen. *J. Immunol.*, **108**:765, 1972.

Hummeler, K., Harris, T. H., Harris, S., and Farber, M. B. Studies on antibody-producing cells. IV. Ultrastructure of plaque forming cells of rabbit lymph. *J. Exp. Med.*, **135**:491, 1972.

Hunter, P., Munro, A., and McConnel, I. Properties of educated T cells for rosette formation and cooperation with B cells. *Nature New Biol.*, **236**:52, 1972.

Katz, D. H., Paul, W. E., and Benacerraf, B. Carrier function in antihapten antibody responses. V. Analysis of cellular events in the enhancement of antibody responses by the "allogenic effect" in DNP-OVA-primed guinea pigs challenged with a heterologous DNP-conjugate. *J. Immunol.*, **107**:1319, 1971.

Kishimoto, T. and Ishizaka, K. Regulation of antibody response *in vitro*. I. Suppression of secondary response by antiimmunoglobulin heavy chains. *J. Immunol.*, **107**:1567, 1971.

Krüger, J. and Gershon, R. K. DNA synthetic response of thymocytes to a variety of antigens. *J. Immunol.*, **108**:581, 1972.

Kurashige, S. and Mitsuhashi, S. Serial passive transfers of immune response by an immune ribonucleic acid preparation. *J. Immunol.*, **108**:1034, 1972.

Lee, S. T., Paraskevas, F., and Israels, L. G. Cell surface associated gamma globulin in lymphocytes. II. The pluripotentiality of mouse spleen lymphocytes. *J. Immunol.*, **107**:1583, 1971.

Levy, R. and Rosenberg, S. A. The early stimulation of protein synthesis in sensitized guinea pig lymph node cells by antigen. *J. Immunol.*, **108**:1073, 1972.

Marchalonis, J. J., Atwell, J. J., and Cone, R. E. Isolation of surface immunoglobulin from lymphocytes from human and murine thymus. *Nature New Biol.*, **235**:241, 1972.

McDonald, H. C., Odstrchel, G., and Maurer, P. H. The influence of carriers on the immune response of rabbits to the synthetic homopolymer poly-(γ-2-N-morpholinylethyl-L-glutamate). *J. Immunol.*, **108**:1690, 1972.

Miller, A., DeLuka, D., Decke, J., Ezzell, R., and Sercarz, E. E. Specific binding of antigen to lymphocytes. *Am. J. Path.*, **65**:451, 1971.

Miller, J. F. A. P., Sprent, J., Basten, A., Warner, N. L., Brietner, J. C. S., Rowland, G., Hamilton, J., Silver, H. and Martin W. J. Cell to cell interaction in the immune response. VII. Requirement for differentiation of thymus derived cells. *J. Exp. Med.* **134**:1266, 1971.

Murphy, M. J., Hay, J. B., Morris, B., and Bessis, M. C. Ultrastructural analysis of antibody synthesis in cells from lymph and lymph nodes. *Am. J. Path.,* **66**:25, 1972.

Pernis, B., Forni, L., and Amante, L. Immunoglobulin spots on the surface of rabbit lymphocytes. *J. Exp. Med.* **132**:1001, 1971.

Raff, M. C. Two distinct populations of peripheral lymphocytes in mice distinguishable by immunofluorescence. *Immunology,* **19**:637, 1970.

Rubin, A. S. and Coons, A. H. Specific heterologous enhancement of immune responses. III. Partial characterization of supernatant material with enhancing antibody. *J. Immunol.,* **108**:1597, 1972.

Sell, S., Lowe, J. A., and Gell, P. G. H. Studies on rabbit lymphocytes *in vitro.* XV. The effect of blocking serum on anti-allotypic lymphocyte transformation. *J. Immunol.,* **108**:674, 1972.

Takahashi, M., Tanigaki, N., Yagi, Y., Moore, G. E., and Pressman, D. Presence of two different immunoglobulin heavy chains in individual cells of established human hematopoietic cell lines. *J. Immunol.,* **100**:1176, 1968.

Taylor, R. B., Duffus, P. H., Raff, M. C., and de Petris, S. Redistribution and pinocytosis of lymphocyte surface immunoglobulin molecules induced by anti-immunoglobulin antibody. *Nature New Biol.,* **233**:225, 1971.

Terres, G., Morrison, S. L., Habicht, G. S., and Stoner, R. D. Appearance of an early "primed state" in mice following the concomitant injection of antigen and specific antiserum. *J. Immunol.,* **108**:1473, 1972.

Weiss, L. *The Cells and Tissues of the Immune System.* Prentice-Hall, Inc., Englewood Cliffs, N.J., 1972.

Chapter 9

Autoimmune Disease

Ranging from disorders with widespread manifestations, such as systemic lupus erythematosus, to fairly organ specific disorders, such as primary hyperthyroidism, nearly every organ exhibits one or more types of chronic inflammatory diseases that appear to be associated with immunity against its own constituents. Evidence for deposition of antiorgan antibodies rests mainly on immunocytochemistry. The presence of immunoglobulin in a location in which it normally is absent, such as in the alveolar basement membrane, is presumptive evidence that an immunologic reaction has taken place in the lesion. The finding does not by itself suggest that the antibodies are etiologically related to the lesion, nor does it suggest that the antibodies are directed against constituents of basement membrane of normal human lung. Evidence for true autoantibodies, though not their role in etiology of a lesion, can be obtained by dissociation of antibodies from the tissue of the diseased host and their specific reattachment to homologous tissue of a normal host as examined with fluorescein-conjugated antiimmunoglobulin. Another method for differentiation between specifically reacting immunoglobulin and nonspecific deposits depends on the restricted heterogeneity of specific antibody compared to that of total host immunoglobulin. A lesser number of L-chain types and H- and L-chain subgroup antigenic specificities in the eluted antibodies than in serum immunoglobulin suggests that the eluted antibodies have been produced by a limited number of lymphoid cells: their formation is, therefore, the result of a specific process. This test does not, however, indicate whether the deposit is antibody reactive with the tissue from which it has been isolated, or with microorganisms infecting such tissues, or whether it is specific antigen-antibody complex formed elsewhere in the host and secondarily deposited in the tissue under examination.

If tissue antigen is in excess, all the antibody produced may be bound to the tissue and none found in circulation. In most of the overt and serious autoimmune diseases, however, a large amount of antibody is also found in circulation. Presence of circulating autoimmune antibodies cannot be postulated in subclinical autoimmune conditions. Demonstration of circulating autoimmune antibodies depends on their reaction with tissue of normal individuals. This again is often demonstrated by indirect immunocytochemistry using biopsies, or autopsy material, or cultured cells of normal organ origin. Other tests include complement fixation with patient's serum and tissue antigen, and agglutination by patient's serum of latex particles, or tanned erythrocytes sensitized with extracts or fragments of normal tissue. In the *immunoglobulin consumption tests* immunoglobulin is eluted from tissue at 56° and reacted with varying dilutions of a standardized antiimmunoglobulin. The unreacted antiimmunoglobulin is then assayed by agglutination of Rh positive, type O erythrocytes sensitized with a nonagglutinating dilution of anti-Rh serum. In some cases the amount of circulating antibodies is high enough to give a precipitin or immunodiffusion test. Direct radioimmunoassay is possible if the antigen reacting with the circulating autoantibodies is known and defined, such as in experimental insulin autoimmunity in which binding with radioiodinated insulin is measured, or in one type of intrinsic factor (gastric) autoimmunity in which the reaction of circulating autoantibodies with intrinsic factor prevents its binding of radiocobalt vitamin B12.

Normally, an individual does not form antibodies to one's own organ constituents or does so in only limited amounts. *Immune tolerance* is acquired in embryonic life and maintained by the persistence of the antigen in later life. Neonatal thymectomy perpetuates the favoring of a tolerance over an immune response into adulthood, even in the absence of large amounts of persisting antigen. Autoimmunity seems to be the replacement of a tolerance response by a hyperimmune response. As long as the mechanism of immune tolerance is poorly understood, proposals for the mechanism of autoimmunity remain somewhat speculative. *Abrogation of immune tolerance, immunologic deficiency,* and *idiotypic antibodies* provide conceivable mechanisms supported by experiments and clinical observation.

ABROGATION OF IMMUNE TOLERANCE

We have already seen that the specificity and avidity of circulating antibody is selected from the specificities and avidities of immunoglobulin receptors on B cells. The size of antigenic determinants responsible for specificity does not exceed a sequence of five to seven amino acids. However, immunogenicity, that is, the amount rather than the specificity of antibody produced, does not depend on such a limited sequence and probably is independent of binding avidity of the B-cell receptor. Immunogenicity as measured by cellular replication depends on a sequence larger than seven amino acids. In an anti*haptenic* response, such as in a response to dinitrophenol, immunogenicity requires a *carrier* much larger in size than the dinitrophenol group, such as provided for example by dinitrophenyl-conjugated hemocyanin. Benacerraff and co-workers have shown that an immune response to hapten is magnified if injection of hapten-carrier conjugate is preceded by injection of carrier devoid of hapten. It has been surmised that the carrier effect is exerted via a helper cell that is distinct from the dinitrophenol-recognizing cell. Apparently, the hapten selects the specificity of immunoglobulin to be formed on a B cell, and the covalently conjugated carrier promotes the helper function through a T cell. Weigle has shown that immunologic tolerance can be abrogated by injection of a cross-reactive antigen. Thus, rabbits tolerant of bovine serum albumin will form antibovine serum albumin following injection of bovine serum albumin coupled with diazotized p-aminophenyl-arsanilic acid. Similarly, immunization with conjugated thyroglobulin abrogates the natural tolerance of thyroglobulin in homologous hosts. The abrogation of the immune response can be explained in the same way as the carrier function in antihaptenic immunity, except that now the specificity recognized by the B cell resides in part of the protein, while the hapten and the remainder of the protein may, perhaps, function as the carrier in a reaction with T cells.

One explanation for the occurrence of autoimmune disease may be provided if it is assumed that the cellular recognition units for protein antigenic determinants remain available throughout the tolerant state, although perhaps masked by combination with persisting antigens. The portion of the protein molecule beyond the antigenic determinant may serve as a carrier for the determinant. Tolerance is perpetuated by the absence of T cells responsive to the carrier portion. Conjugation of the protein with arsanilic acid alters the carrier portion of the native antigen. This alteration may evoke a different group of T cells, thus, helping towards completion of an immune response to the native antigen. Provocation of an autoimmune response by such a mechanism requires that an extraneous stimulus alters organ constituents to which normally a host is tolerant. The natural histories of several of the autoimmune disorders discussed below provide such stimuli either in the form of fulminating antecedent infections or in the form of slow viruses. These stimuli may produce altered organ constituents either by covalent binding of infectious products, or by membrane fusion of viral envelope with host cells (page 94), or by incorporation of viral determinants into the genome of the host cell.

An alternative explanation for abrogation of tolerance and establishment of autoimmunity can be arrived at by solubility considerations of the antigen alone. Soluble antigens are more tolerogenic than immunogenic, while aggregated antigens are more immunogenic (page 209). In a normal environment an autologous antigen, such thyroglobulin, does not become aggregated and, thus, tolerance of this antigen is maintained. However, if one immunizes with arsanilic acid-conjugated thyroglobulin, antibodies to the arsanilate hapten form antigen-antibody complexes with the conjugated thyroglobulin. Conjugated thyroglobulin possesses antigenic determinants in common with native thyroglobulin. Thus, native determinants become aggregated, and an immune response ensues.

IMMUNOLOGIC DEFICIENCY

H. Fudenberg emphasizes the association of "adult onset" hypogammaglobulinemia, a genetic disorder, with a high incidence of autoimmune disease and of malignancy. A genetically determined T-cell defect may only be partial in that it affords only the response to few specific antigens, such as staphylococcal antigens or a single synthetic polypeptide antigen. As a result antigens could accumulate that alter autologous proteins and abrupt the preexisting tolerance of these proteins. Similarly, specific deficiencies may permit proliferation of slow viruses that insidiously could abrupt a preexisting organ immune tolerance. Also antinuclear antibodies, discussed later, normally absent from circulation because of immune tolerance, could be induced by viral DNA and RNA via a mechanism reminiscent of the induction of antibodies to single stranded DNA or RNA by carrier-conjugated bases.

IDIOTYPIC ANTIBODIES

Mouse plasmocytoma protein 315 (a myeloma IgA) binds dinitrophenol with a high degree of specificity. The protein bears BALB/c allotype on its α-chain. S. Shirisinha and H. Eisen find that, nevertheless, immunization of BALB/c mice produces antibodies against the protein 315. Binding of the antibodies and the protein is inhbited by dinitrophenol. Hence, the antigenic determinants of protein 315 that evoke antibodies in the BALB/c mice are in or near its specific combining sites: the antibodies are idiotypic. Animals are normally tolerant of idiotypic and allotypic determinants of their own proteins. Indeed, no antibodies are evoked in BALB/c mice against determinants of protein 315 except those at the specific combining sites. Idiotypic determinants in the immunized host's own immunoglobulins are, apparently, present in too small quantities to induce tolerance. Hence, injection of the large amounts of these determinants provided by isologous immunoglobulins, such as protein 315 (the product of a single clone of plasma cells), may provoke an immune response. Similarly, production of large amounts of antibodies in an overwhelming infection may provide immunoglobulins of restricted heterogeneity that in turn could induce autoimmune idiotypic antibodies, i.e., antiimmunoglobulin autoimmunity.

PATHOGENICITY

Tissue damage in autoimmune disease is due to delayed hypersensitivity or to cytotoxicity. *Delayed hypersensitivity* is manifested by infiltration into tissue of lymphoid, mononuclear, and plasma cells and is proved by transfer of the specific lesion to isogeneic hosts by lymphoid cells. Another test is provided by inhibition of macrophage (capillary tube) migration by lymphocytes from the autoimmune donor in the presence of the antigen responsible for autoimmunity. The presence of specific immunoglobulin in the lesion or circulation of the diseased animal or patient may be of diagnostic value but has no bearing on the production of the delayed sensitivity lesion and, indeed, may inhibit it.

The *cytotoxic mechanism* of pathogenesis in autoimmunity is due to reaction of large amounts of antigen and antibody. As a result, antigen-antibody complexes deposit both in the organs of the primary lesion as well as in the capillary beds of distant locations, such as the renal glomeruli. If these complexes consist of antigen and specific IgG or IgM, they fix complement leading to a cytotoxic reaction with the cells on which they are deposited.

In the individual experimental and clinical autoimmune syndromes described below, we will encounter preponderance of hypersensitivity or cytotoxicity mechanisms. We will also encounter examples that support the tolerance abrogation or the immune deficiency mechanism of etiology.

GLOMERULONEPHRITIS

Immunofluorescence of affected glomeruli with anti-IgG reveal two patterns of localization. A linear deposit (Fig. 9-1) is characteristic of Goodpasture's disease, a rapidly fatal illness manifested by hemoptysis, anemia, hematuria, renal failure, and pulmonary hemorrhages, and restricted pathologically to lungs and kidneys. Linear deposits are also found in less fulminating instances, such as in a large number of subacute and chronic glomerulonephritides of adults. Granular deposits, that is, discrete irregular and lumpy deposits (Fig. 9-2), are characteristic of the

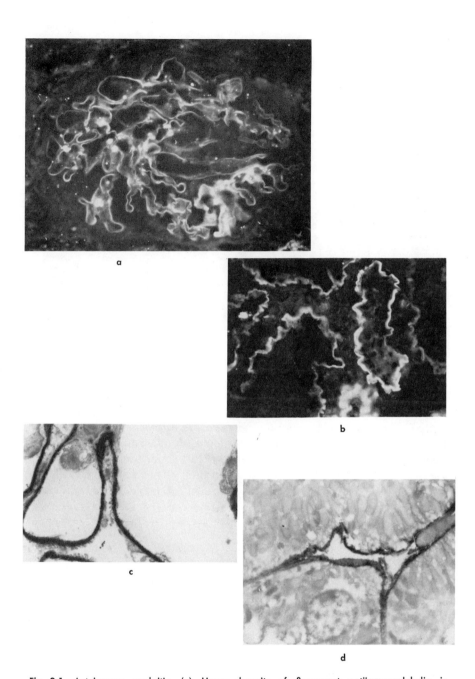

Fig. 9-1 Autoimmune nephritis. (a) Linear deposits of fluorescent antiimmunoglobulin in glomerular basement membrane in human glomerulonephritis. X800. (b) Linear deposits of fluorescent antiimmunoglobulin in tubular basement membrane in human renal allograft. X700. (c) Localization of glomerular basement membrane in nephrotoxic nephritis of the rat. Unlabeled antibody enzyme method. X5,000. (d) Localization of tubular basement membrane in nephrotoxic nephritis of the rat. Unlabeled antibody enzyme method. X4,000. From the work of Giuseppe A. Andres.

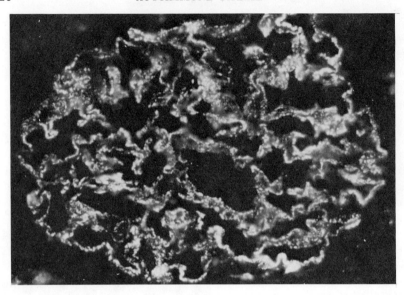

Fig. 9-2 Immunofluorescence profile of immune complex glomerulonephritis: granular deposits of fluorescent antiimmunoglobulin in glomerular basement membrane. X700. From the work of Giuseppe A. Andres.

nephritis following β hemolytic streptococcal infections (such as tonsillitis, scarlet fever or pyodermia), of the nephritis associated with acute and subacute bacterial endocarditis, and lupus erythematosus, and of the nephrosis accompanying quartan malaria. The lesions in both linear and granular immunofluorescence reveal infiltration of polymorphonuclear leukocytes and absence of mononuclear cells. This excludes delayed sensitivity as the mechanism of renal pathogenesis.

GOODPASTURE'S SYNDROME

The immunoglobulin revealed by immunofluorescence in Goodpasture's syndrome can be eluted from glomeruli or alveoli by treatment at pH 3.2 at 37° for two hours. The eluted material binds specifically with human alveolar and renal tissue as revealed by immunofluorescence. The material fails to bind with other tissues. The eluate also binds with glomerular basement membrane of the mouse and other species but not with alveolar basement membrane of the mouse. The findings suggest that the immunoglobulin bound in Goodpasture's syndrome is an autoantibody or a group of autoantibodies cross-reactive with lung and kidney. The cross-reactivity is species specific. At least some of the antibodies are organ specific, but not species specific; that is, they react with basement membrane of the kidneys in many species, but not with basement membrane of other organs. The antibodies are not homogeneous: in one patient described by T. Poskitt *post mortem* glomerular tissue is stained by anti-IgG$_1$, anti-IgG$_2$, and anti-IgG$_4$ but not by anti-IgG$_3$. Hence, the antibodies have not been produced by a restricted clone of immunocompetent cells. Their specificities may not be identical, and it is feasible that some types are cross-reactive with human lung, while others are cross-reactive with mouse kidney. The failure to find IgG$_3$ is additional evidence that the IgG is deposited in the basement membrane as a result of an antigen-antibody reaction, and not merely resorbed from serum as a nonspecific sequella of another renal lesion that may have increased accessibility of the basement membrane to circulating proteins.

Sometimes complement can be revealed in the affected kidney by direct or indirect immunofluorescence with anti-C1q, anti-C4, or anti-C3. Whether this can be demonstrated or not, the antibody eluted from glomeruli fixes complement with basement membrane antigen *in vitro*. Moreover, immunoglobulins eluted from affected kidneys and localized specifically in the glomerular basement membranes of injected mice, sheep, and squirrel monkeys, cause in the latter two species fulminating glomerulonephritis with evidence of glomerular deposition of complement components.

The circulation of patients with linear deposit type of nephritis does not reveal antikidney antibodies. However, Lerner, Glassrock, and Dixon observed that following nephrectomy prior to renal transplantation there is a rapid rise in circulating antikidney antibodies. After transplantation the circulating antibodies disappear again, being bound by the transplant along with complement. Apparently, renal tissue acts as a sink for a large amount of autoimmune antibody absorbing all detectable antibody from circulation. The large amount of antigen supplied by any tissue in autoimmune diseases may, thus, evoke a massive antigen-antibody reaction capable of the close packing of IgG on the tissue that is necessary for fixation of complement.

The massive antigen-antibody reaction observed in Goodpasture's syndrome, the ability to transfer the nephritis to experimental animals by eluted antibodies (rather than by cells) and the fixation of complement, suggests that the antibody observed by immunofluorescence in this disease is responsible for its pathogenesis. The damage to tissue is cytotoxic via complement. Delayed sensitivity (cellular immunity) does not play an important role in the pathogenesis.

Injection of renal basement membrane material produces linear immunofluorescence deposit nephritis in heterologous as well as homologous hosts. This reproduction of autoimmune nephritis in experimental animals suggests but does not prove an autoimmune etiology of the spontaneous disease in man. Neither does it permit distinction between a tolerance breakdown or immunologic deficiency etiology of the disease. The fact that experimental nephritis has been produced by injection of lung tissue and that injection of kidney tissue does not induce a pulmonary disease may perhaps suggest, by inference, that in Goodpasture's syndrome the lung lesion is primary. The course of the disease in which initial symptoms are confined to the lungs seems to support this assumption.

IMMUNE COMPLEX DISEASE

When a large amount of foreign protein is injected into an experimental animal, renal pathology does not result if the immune response is efficient or if the animal is immune tolerant. Transient renal pathology, as revealed by granular deposits on immunofluorescence with antiimmunoglobulin, results only if the immune response is moderate. In the case of an efficient response, antibody is in excess, and the antigen precipitates. The precipitates are taken up by the reticuloendothelial system, and no renal pathology ensues. However, if the immune response is moderate the antigen-antibody complexes are formed in antigen excess. These complexes are caught in the filtering system of the kidneys and can be detected by immunofluorescence. Their predilection for the kidney is apparently due to the large circulatory volume passing through the renal arteries and to direct accessibility of the glomerular basement membrane to the capillary lumen via breaks in the endothelial surface (page 67). Complexes of three antigen and two specific IgG molecules, and larger antigen-IgG complexes, fix complement as they contain more than one IgG subunits (page 11). When such complexes localize at the renal basement membrane, damage to surrounding tissue results.

If the immune response is poor, no antibodies form, or their amounts are so small that they combine with antigen in such high antigen excess that the resulting complexes consist of two antigen and one antibody molecule. Complexes of two antigens and one IgG molecule do not fix complement. They cause no cytotoxic pathology.

Complement disappears from circulation during the development of kidney lesions after injection of antigen into experimental animals. The lesions mimic *serum sickness* of man in all respects. The renal pathology is *transitory,* and recovery is complete.

Circulating antigen-IgG complexes that are too small for elimination by phagocytosis do not in themselves become entrapped in the filtering system of the glomeruli despite breaks in the endothelial surface. Entrapment only occurs once capillary permeability is increased. P. M. Henson and C. G. Chochrane find that glomerulonephritis develops only in rabbits that form specific IgE in addition to IgG after injection of antigen. In the presence of antigen basophil-bound IgE (page 13) releases an intermediate that clumps platelets and mediates liberation of vasoactive amines from the aggregated platelets. The resulting increased vascular permeability appears to be the cause of entrapment of the cytotoxic, soluble antigen-IgG complexes (the basophil intermediate appears to be independent of basophil histamine and degranulation).

Progressive renal lesions characterized by granular immunofluorescence may appear as sequellae or accompanying manifestations of severe infections or severe, chronic autoimmune diseases. Experimental immune thyroiditis (page 225) is normally confined to a purely thyroid pathology. However, if the afflicted thyroid is damaged by radioiodine, there is extensive leakage of thyroglobulin from the gland into circulation. Circulating complexes of thyroglobulin and autoimmune antibodies form, and progressive glomerulonephritis ensues.

The glomerulonephritis that follows β hemolytic streptococcal infection reveals granular deposits by immunofluorescence after reaction with anti-IgG, anticomplement as well as antiserum against type 12 streptococcal products.

One may ask why soluble antigen-antibody complexes entrapped in the glomeruli in chronic immune complex disease should persist so long in this location as part of a chronic, often progressive lesion. Soluble complexes can exist only in the presence of excess of antigen. In most antigen-antibody systems the required excess is large. Complexes may well be entrapped in a soluble state, while the concentration of circulating antigen is high. Upon subsequent immune elimination of circulating antigen, the entrapped complexes reequilibriate by release of antigen and formation of complexes of lower antigen-antibody ratios. If the antibody avidity is high, such as in chronic immune complex disease, the reequilibriated complexes form immune precipitates and are revealed as persisting lesions by immunofluorescence. On the other hand, if the avidity is low, such as in serum sickness type of lesions produced by single immunizing injections, dissociation of antigen from the complexes continues to completion and releases the entrapped antibody as well. The lesions demonstrated by immunofluorescence are transitory.

The size of circulating antigen-antibody complexes responsible for renal lesions is usually measured by gradient sedimentation using radiolabeled antigens. The serum is placed as a zone on top of the gradient. During sedimentation, complex moves towards the bottom of the gradient, away from the free antigen that remains close to the top. As a result, the sedimenting complex reequilibriates continually releasing antigen that is assayed by radioactivity determinations (see also pages 137 and 139 and Fig. 6-5). A complex of low avidity releases antigen faster and, thus, falsely appears lighter than a complex of high avidity. Hence, correlation of pathology with size of complexes as determined by zonal sedimentation should be evaluated with caution.

SLOW VIRUSES AND CANCER VIRUSES

Mice of the New Zealand Black (NZB) strain develop autoimmune hemolytic anemia spontaneously. This is confirmed by the direct antiglobulin Coombs test in which binding of immunoglobulin to erythrocytes is demonstrated by their agglutination with anti-IgG. Certain hybrid progeny strains of NZB mice develop, however, a fulminating glomerulonephritis and circulating antinuclear antibodies associated with edema, ascitis, pleural effusion, pulmonary edema, and gastrointestinal hemorrhage. The syndrome mimics in many respects lupus erythematosus in man, discussed below. These mice, like several other mouse strains, harbor Gross leukemia virus (page 102) and express virus group (internal virion) antigens (page 146) throughout life in extracts of normal organs, as well as in malignant lymphomas developing spontaneously with high frequency. The Gross soluble antigen (GSA) is one of the nonvirion antigens specified by the Gross leukemia virus. R. Mellors found that the production of GSA coincides closely with the appearance of a positive, direct antiglobulin Coombs test. Unlike other strains of mice bearing the Gross leukemia viruses, NZB mice are not tolerant to Gross antigens. The break in tolerance, apparently, is the starting point for the massive antibody production, resulting in the lupus erythematosus-like syndrome. Thus, autoimmune disease in this case is, apparently, caused by a genetic immunologic deficiency. The tolerance itself may have been abrogated by membrane fusion (page 94) with autologous cell surface antigen.

Aleutian mink disease is caused by a slow virus and manifested by plasmacytosis, hypergammaglobulinemia, and glomerulonephritis. Autoimmunity is demonstrated by a positive Coombs test and by anti-DNA antibodies. H. Cho and D. G. Ingram were able to show that a specific Aleutian mink disease antigen in spleen, kidney, and liver is masked by antibodies 13 days after infection. Acid treatment removes the antibodies and makes the antigen available for serologic tests with antibody. I. C. Pan, K. Tsai, and L. Karstad have demonstrated by immunofluorescence the presence of immunoglobulin and complement in the renal glomerular capillary walls.

AUTOIMMUNE THYROIDITIS

Antibodies reactive with thyroglobulin and sometimes with two other thyroid antigens are found in the circulation of patients afflicted with lymphatic thyroiditis. The antibodies are usually IgG, occasionally IgM, or IgA. The amount and frequency of detection of antibodies apparently parallels severity of the various forms of lymphocytic thyroiditis. As much as 19 mg/ml of precipitating antithyroglobulin has been isolated from a case of a fibrous variant of goiterous, diffuse, lymphocytic thyroiditis (Hashimoto's disease). Circulating antibodies can also be demonstrated with high frequency in severe atrophic thyroiditis (myxedema). Mild atrophic thyroiditis that is a common disorder, exhibiting mild hypothyroidism, is occasionally associated with circulating antibodies in low levels. Pathologic diagnosis depends primarily on immunofluorescence of thyroid tissue with antiimmunoglobulin conjugate. Immunofluorescence also reveals complement bound in the lesion. The circulating antibodies are cytotoxic to cultured thyroid cells. These are, of course, properties expected of IgG and IgM. The findings are consistent with a cytotoxic etiology of autoimmune thyroiditis but do not prove it as the main mechanism.

The lymphoid infiltration would suggest a hypersensitivity etiology. However, a hypersensitivity mechanism has been proven only in thyroiditis induced experimentally by the immunization with thyroglobulin in complete Freund's adjuvants (water in oil emulsion of antigen and mycobacteria with or without *Bordetella pertussis*).

R. Bucsi and H. Strausser report that neonatally thymectomized and sham-operated mice form on immunization with thyroglobulin and adjuvants similar levels of circulating antibodies, but in the thymectomized animals the thyroiditis as evaluated by lymphoid infiltration is greatly depressed. Neonatal thymectomy depresses the development of cell-mediated hypersensitive immune responses. Circulating antibodies alone are apparently unable to cause thyroiditis in experimental animals.

Papillary thyroid cancer is often associated with focal or diffuse lymphoid infiltrations. About 50% of patients with thyroid cancer give a positive test for circulating antibodies to thyroid.

The Buffalo strain of rats possesses unusual sensitivity towards the production of thyroiditis by immunization with thyroglobulin. 3-methylcholanthrene, a carcinogen, also induces thyroiditis in these rats. D. Silverman and N. Rose find in both forms of thyroiditis circulating autoantibodies to thyroid giving positive indirect immunofluorescence with normal rat thyroid. Methylcholanthrene has a direct effect on the thyroid. It is conceivable, therefore, that autoimmune thyroiditis develops secondarily to damage to the thyroid. The findings suggest caution in inferring an analogy between experimental thyroiditis induced by immunization and autoimmune thyroiditis observed clinically. The experimental thyroiditis requires adjuvants for immunization, a procedure known to evoke cell-mediated immunity. The tissue damage in the experimentally induced disease is expected, therefore, to be due to hypersensitivity.

It is conceivable that in clinical, lymphocytic thyroiditis the tissue damage is primary along with the lymphoid infiltration. Secondary release of thyroglobulin and other thyroid antigens, native or modified by the primary disease process, then might evoke a circulating antibody response. In this sequence of events, the damage by antibodies if any may be only cytotoxic, while infiltration of lymphocytes in the thyroid could be unrelated to autoimmunity altogether.

Primary hyperthyroidism (Grave's disease) is caused by an overstimulation of the thyroid. The thyroid-stimulating substance is, however, not thyrotropic hormone, but an immunoglobulin. Its thyroid-stimulating activity rests in its Fab portion and, hence, is probably due to reaction with antigen. Thyroid tissue removes thyroid-stimulating activity from serum. The thyroid-stimulating substance can be adsorbed onto a microsomal fraction of thyroid tissue and eluted from it at pH 3.5.

GASTRIC AUTOIMMUNITY

Pernicious anemia is a macrocytic anemia associated with a gastric secretory defect (lack of "intrinsic factor") and changes in the nervous system and characterized by responsiveness to vitamin B12. Two lines of evidence suggest autoimmunity in pernicious anemia. One is the presence in pernicious anemia serum of antibodies reacting with the cytoplasm of the gastric parietal cells, and the other is the presence of antibodies reacting with intrinsic factor. Also, antiparietal cell antibodies within the parietal cells, are demonstrated by immunofluorescence of pernicious anemia gastric mucosa with conjugated anti-IgG. Complement is fixed in the lesion as shown by immunofluorescence with conjugated anticomplement. Lymphoid germinal centers are seen in the gastric mucosa. It is conceivable that the autoimmune lesion is primary leading to atrophy of the gastric mucosa and failure of secretion of acid, intrinsic factor and pepsin.

Several sera of patients with pernicious anemia who had never received hog intrinsic factor neutralize the biologic activity of intrinsic factor. Antibodies that react close to the vitamin B12 combining site of intrinsic factor block its reaction with vitamin B12 and can be assayed by binding tests of radioiodinated vitamin B12 with intrinsic factor. Other antibodies react at a site distant to the binding site for vitamin B12. These antibodies are assayed by precipitation with half saturation in ammonium sulfate. Radiocobalt vitamin B12 bound on intrinsic factor remains in the supernatant, while radiocobalt vitamin B12 bound with intrinsic factor-antibody complex is precipitated. The antiintrinsic factor antibodies do not fix complement and are not revealed by immunofluorescence. They are probably not cytotoxic. Their pathogenicity resides in inactivation of intrinsic factor.

There is a high frequency association of pernicious anemia and autoimmune thyroiditis (lymphocytic thyroiditis as well as primary hyperthyroidism). Both kinds of disorders are characterized by highly organ-specific antibodies. Cell destruction is also limited to the organs affected. Nonorganspecific antibodies, such as antinuclear antibodies, are only rarely observed in these disorders. On the other hand, in such generalized autoimmune disorders as lupus erythematosus, there is only a low incidence of organspecific antibodies.

Lupus Erythematosus

Lupus erythematosus is a progressive, multiorgan disease initiating with articular and cutaneous involvement and presenting during the course of the disease, in addition to these manifestations, fever, renal, pleuritic, pericarditic, and neuropsychiatric manifestations, along with anemia, leukopenia, and elevated immunoglobulins. The disease may be self-limited, or it may be relentlessly progressive, nephritis being often diagnosed within one year after initial symptoms. Renal failure is the usual cause of death.

Characteristic of lupus erythematosus is the presence of serum antibodies reactive with the patient's cells, with cells from normal individuals or even with cells of animal origin. At least five different groups of antigens that react with the sera of various patients are described by E. Tan. Some patients' sera react with only one of these antigen groups. Others react with many. However, all lupus erythematosus sera possess antibodies that are reactive with widely distributed antigens, that is antigens that are neither organ-specific nor species-specific. DNA is characteristically such an antigen. Possessing only four nucleotide determinants, the number of antigens that can be specified by a DNA sequence is much less than the number of antigens specified by a peptide incorporating permutations of 22 amino acids. Consequently, antibodies to proteins are likely to be highly specific, and diseases with autoimmune antibodies to proteins are usually restricted to few organs. Thus, autoimmune thyroiditis with antibodies to thyroglobulin is usually manifested in the thyroid only. On the other hand, in lupus erythematosus with antibodies to DNA, there is no organ or even species

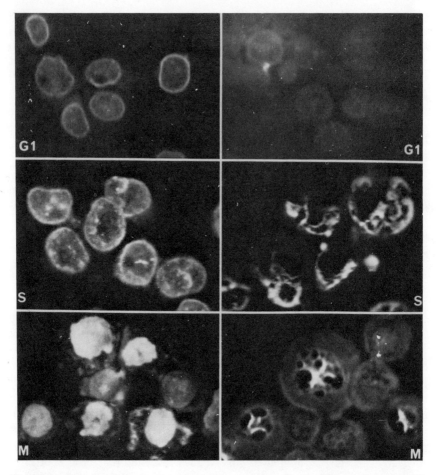

Fig. 9-3 Indirect immunofluorescence of nuclear macromolecules in different phases of WIL$_2$ cells (continuously growing diploid lymphocytes derived from the spleen of a patient with hereditary spherocytosis). G1, pre-DNA synthesis phase; S, DNA synthesis phase; M, mitotic phase of cell division. X900. Left panel is the staining pattern with lupus erythematosus serum monospecific for native DNA, right panel with lupus erythematosus serum monospecific for single stranded DNA. From E. M. Tan and R. A. Lerner, *J. Mol. Biol.*, **68**:107, 1972.

specificity of reaction. Consequently, clinical manifestations are widespread and involve multiple organ systems. Diagnosis of lupus erythematosus depends on reaction of patient's serum with cells, such as cultures of WIL$_2$ cells, and immunocytochemical detection of this reaction with antiimmunoglobulin (Figs. 9-3 to 9-5).

Five groups of antigen are described that react with lupus erythematosus serum by indirect immunofluorescence: native DNA, single stranded DNA, nucleoprotein, an unidentified protein antigenically not dependent

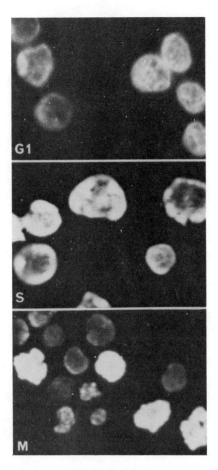

Fig. 9-4 WIL$_2$ cells similar to Fig. 9-3. The cells were treated with lupus erythematosus serum monospecific for desoxyribonucleoprotein. From E. M. Tan and R. A. Lerner, *J. Mol. Biol.*, **68**:107, 1972.

on nucleic acid determinants, and a nuclear ribonucleoprotein. Patients' sera may contain antibodies to one or several of these groups of antigens as apparent by the number of immunodiffusion lines formed with the respective groups of antigens and by lines of identity or diversity among sera from different patients.

Antiserum to native DNA gives a line of identity with native DNA, sonicated, and heat-denatured DNA. With WIL$_2$ cells made monophasic by arrest of mitosis with colchicine and subsequent release from arrest, this antiserum stains by indirect immunofluorescence only the nuclear rim in the preDNA synthesis phase (G1) of the cells (Fig. 9-3). In the S-phase (DNA synthesis phase) the rim staining becomes stronger and, in addition,

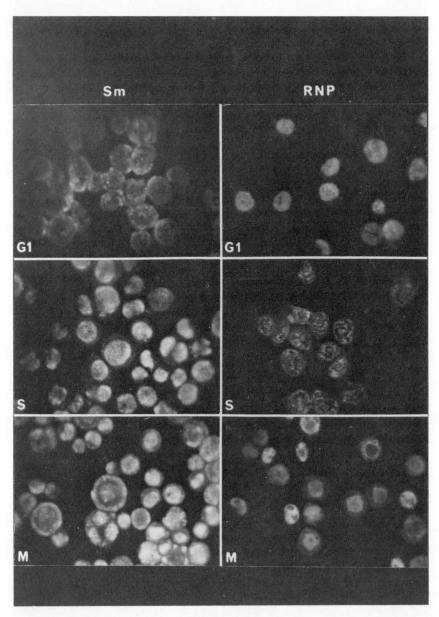

Fig. 9-5 Similar to cells in Figs. 9-3 and 9-4. The left panel shows the pattern of distribution of indirect immunofluorescence with lupus erythematosus serum monospecific for the Sm antigen. Sm is in the nucleus and the cytoplasm. The cytoplasmic staining is most clearly demonstrated in the G1 and M phases. The right panel shows the pattern of distribution of indirect immunofluorescence with lupus erythematosus serum monospecific for ribonucleoprotein. Ribonucleoprotein is exclusively nuclear in the G1 phase. In the S phase ribonucleoprotein is primarily nuclear with a speckled and diffuse morphology differing from that seen with anti-Sm. In the M phase ribonucleoprotein is more predominently nuclear than Sm antigen. X450. From J. D. Northway and E. M. Tan, *Clin. Immunol. Immunopath.*, 1:140, 1972.

lumps of staining project into the central nuclear region from the periphery. In the M-phase (mitosis) the whole nucleus is stained strongly as well as what appears to be some cytoplasmic DNA.

Antiserum to single stranded DNA is identified by a precipitin line with heat denatured DNA that is absent with native or sonicated DNA. These antibodies yield no immunofluorescence in the G1 phase, but produce strong staining in the S-phase, especially along the nuclear membrane. The M-phase also reveals the presence of some single stranded DNA.

Some antisera react by immunodiffusion with a soluble, nuclear material sedimenting at S19 or higher. The reaction disappears if the material is digested with trypsin or with DNAase but not with RNAase. Thus, the serum seems to react with an antigenic determinant resulting from combination of DNA with a protein. That this protein is a histone is demonstrated by the appearance of a precipitin line upon diffusion of this serum against DNA mixed with histone *in vitro*. Immunofluorescence with lupus erythematosus serum monospecific to DNA-histone complex gives homogeneous nuclear staining in the G1 phase, becoming stronger in the S-phase and roughly indicating chromosomal shapes in the M-phase (Fig. 9-4). Absence of cytoplasmic staining in the M-phase suggests that cytoplasmic DNA is not associated with histone.

Another antigen reactive with some lupus erythematosus sera, called Sm antigen by E. Tan, is an acidic protein of about 100,000 molecular weight found by immunofluorescence in the nucleus and to a lesser extent in the cytoplasm. Sm antigen is revealed in all phases of cell division.

The fifth antigen is apparently a nuclear ribonucleoprotein that cross-reacts with the Sm antigen (spur formation on immunodiffusion). The two antigens have different distributions on immunofluorescence in synchronized cells (Fig. 9-5).

Single or double stranded DNA as well as RNA or histone are poor antigens. Apparently, tolerance to these antigens is found in most species. The similarity of structure of the polynucleotides per unit length within the confines of the maximum size of an antigenic determinant (page 215), and perhaps the richness of basic groups in histone may insure that tolerance is not species specific. Consequently, it is not possible to simulate lupus erythematosus in experimental animals, even when complete Freund's adjuvants are given with heterologous antigen. This contrasts with the organ-specific thyroiditis or organ-specific encephalitis that can be produced by immunization with thyroglobulin or with nervous tissue and Freund's adjuvants. The strong tolerance normally encountered against antigens reactive with lupus erythematosus serum is undoubtedly related to their ubiquitousness. However, once antibodies to these antigens are formed the autoimmune reaction is widespread, and the manifestations of the disease involve many organ systems.

Slow virus infection is sometimes suspected as cause of lupus erythematosus. It is implicit in this assumption that part of the nucleotide sequence in these viruses is sufficiently different from mammalian polynucleotides, as to be recognized as immunogens or, alternatively, that the viral nucleic acids are complexed with a protein carrier other than a histone, thus making the nucleotide antigenic by a hapten carrier mechanism.

Nephritis is the most serious manifestation of lupus erythematosus. This is an immune complex nephritis characterized by granular immunofluorescence deposits with antibodies against IgG, third component of complement and nucleoprotein.

Lupus erythematosus is characterized by frequent, febrile exacerbations and remissions. During remissions, the patient's serum usually contains free antibodies. During exacerbations, the serum contains excess antigen. It is during these periods that antigen is released, reacting with all available antibody and exacerbating the deposits of immune complexes in the kidneys [we recall that serum sickness does not occur when excess antibody is found in circulation (page 222)]. Serum sickness manifests itself when soluble antigen-antibody complexes of smaller size, formed in antigen excess, are caught in the subendothelial filtering system of the renal glomeruli. Lupus erythematosus is a cytotoxic disease in which damage to cells appears to be mediated via complement and not via the cellular mechanism of delayed sensitivity.

IMMUNOLOGIC SKIN DISEASES

Indirect immunofluorescence with labeled antihuman immunoglobulin is particularly useful in the diagnosis of bullous skin disease. In pemphigus there is widespread blistering of skin and mucous membranes. The untreated disease is always fatal.

The lesion is characterized by acantholysis (solvation of the matrix that cements together the cells of the stratified squamous epithelium). Indirect immunofluorescence with antiimmunoglobulin reveals the outlines of the stratified squamous cells. Immunofluorescence does not reveal complement in the lesion. Circulating antibodies are specific to the polysaccharide cement substance of the stratified squamous epithelium.

The absence of localization of complement suggests that the lesion is not due to cytotoxicity of the antibodies. However, the occasional finding of circulating antibodies prior to development of the lesion and the usefulness of corticosteroid and immunosuppressive therapy do suggest an autoimmune mechanism in the pathogenesis of the disease. There is a high frequency association between pemphigus and myasthenia gravis.

In bullous pemphigoid, a more benign disease, the blisters are subepidermal. Mortality is 5%. There are no free floating cells. Immunofluorescence demonstrates circulating antibodies to normal basement membrane. Complement is fixed in the lesion.

AUTOIMMUNE LIVER DISEASE

Primary biliary cirrhosis, active chronic hepatitis, and certain cases of cryptogenic cirrhosis give rise to circulating antibodies with antinuclear, antimitochondrial, and antismooth muscle specificities. Although antimitochondrial antibodies are particularly diagnostic for primary biliary cirrhosis and smooth muscle antibodies for active chronic hepatitis, the simultaneous occurrence of these antibodies in all three diseases and their conspicuous absence in other liver disorders, such as alcoholic cirrhosis or chronic persistent hepatitis associated with Australia (hepatitis virus) antigen, suggests that the three disorders are related. Indeed, liver biopsies have been obtained that contain both, areas of primary biliary cirrhosis (characterized by necrosis of bile ducts) and areas of active chronic hepatitis (necrosis of hepatocytes). In the lesion of both diseases, there is mononuclear cell infiltration with accumulation into lymphoid follicles. Both diseases may progress to advanced cirrhosis with the histology of cryptogenic cirrhosis. About 90% of sera of patients with primary biliary cirrhosis give granular, indirect immunofluorescence with the cytoplasm of normal cells. These reactions are neither organ nor species specific and are especially prominent in cells rich in mitochondria. The reactive antigen is a lipoprotein component of the mitochondrial inner membrane.

Antibody reactive with smooth muscle is detected by indirect immunofluorescence in about 70% of patients with active chronic hepatitis (juvenile hepatitis). Again the reaction exhibits no organ specificity.

In line with the lack of organ specificity of the antimitochondrial, antismooth muscle, and antinuclear antibodies in these diseases, it is not surprising that active, chronic hepatitis is frequently associated with other autoimmune manifestations, such as thyroiditis, ulcerative colitis, diabetes, necrotizing dermal arteriolitis, renal tubular lesions, fever, arthralgia, and other manifestations of lupus erythematosus. A usually mild glomerulonephritis found in active chronic hepatitis may be a cytotoxic (immune complex) manifestation. The lymphoid cell infiltration may be an expression of delayed sensitivity. Release of antigen from the liver as a result of a primary disease process is probably not etiologically related to autoimmune liver disease, since the characteristic antibodies are absent or rarely present in other liver diseases that present similar histology (such as cholestatic drug jaundice, obstructive cholangitis, viral hepatitis, and alcoholic cirrhosis).

Some forms of chronic, persistent hepatitis and of cirrhosis are associated with the presence of large amounts of Australia antigen and the presence in the circulation of specific antibodies. Immune complex nephritis is sometimes found. It is a heteroimmune nephritis. Interestingly, even such extensive, perhaps necrotizing Australia antigen-antibody reaction in the liver, apparently does not initiate production of *auto*-immune antibodies.

ULCERATIVE COLITIS

Nonspecific, ulcerative colitis is characterized by dehaustration and ulceration of the mucosal and submucosal layers, mainly in the large intestine. The chronic disease is manifested by bloody diarrhea, abdominal pain, loss of weight, and anemia. Patients' sera contain IgM antibodies that are found by indirect immunofluorescence to react with an antigen in the cytoplasm of the mucus-producing cells of the colonic mucosa. The antigen is chemically related to bacterial mucopolysaccharide. Occasionally, the reaction with colonic antigen has been abolished by absorption with a phenol-water extract of *E. coli*. Complement levels in patients with ulcerative colitis are normal. Ulcerative colitis serum is not cytotoxic to colon cells in tissue culture. However, leukocytes, presumably lymphocytes, from a patient with ulcerative colitis cause inflammatory reactions when injected into his own rectal mucosa. The evidence seems to favor hypersensitivity as the disease-producing mechanism, while circulating antibodies seem to play no role in the formation of the lesion.

Normally, the predominant immunoglobulin in the lymphoid cells of the lamina propria of the human rectal mucosa is IgA. Conceivably, but not certainly the secretory immunoglobulin may have a protective role, perhaps, as a first barrier towards invasion of the mucosa by intestinal microorganisms. S. Kraft and associates using fluorescein isothiocyanate-conjugated anti-IgA find that in ulcerative colitis the number of IgA-containing cells is reduced, and the distribution of the cells that do contain IgA is focal, thereby, leaving large areas devoid of IgA-bearing cells. The IgA is found in extracellular interstitial spaces below the mucosal surface, a localization not seen in normal subjects.

As the pathogenesis of ulcerative colitis is probably via delayed sensitivity and as the associated circulating anticolon antibodies are exclusively or primarily IgM, one may raise the question whether deficiency of IgA is not related to pathogenesis. Perhaps IgA deficiency leads to increasing invasiveness of intestinal microorganisms that in turn taxes an overactive response of other immune systems, such as IgM-producing cells and cells of delayed sensitivity. The primary antigen in such a mechanism would have to be related to a constituent of an intestinal microorganism. This sequence of pathogenesis would appear to illustrate immunologic deficiency as an etiologic factor in an autoimmune disease.

MYASTHENIA GRAVIS

Abnormal fatigability, rapid exhaustion, and loss of voluntary muscle strength are the chief manifestations of myasthenia gravis. Partial restoration of muscle strength with anticholinesteratic drugs incriminates the myoneural junction as the main site of the affliction. The bulk of circulating antibodies that are found in myasthenia gravis react by indirect immunofluorescence, not with the myoneural junction, but with the alternate striations of normal or myasthenic skeletal muscles.

In some cases of myasthenia gravis, a large number of germinal centers are seen in the thymus. Whether or not germinal centers are seen, thymectomy often induces remission of the muscular symptoms. Interestingly, V. Perlo and co-workers find that thymectomy in cases without germinal centers induces early remission, while in cases with many germinal centers remission is delayed. The demonstration that muscle cells and thymic epithelial cells share a cross-reacting antigen, and the frequent association of myasthenia gravis with thymoma may incriminate the thymus as the primary organ of pathogenesis. The role of the thymus in the disease and the effect of thymectomy suggests cellular hypersensitivity as the mechanism of pathogenesis.

RHEUMATOID ARTHRITIS

It is uncertain whether rheumatoid arthritis is an autoimmune or heteroimmune disease. Rheumatoid factor that is seen in the circulation of the majority of patients is an IgM reactive with the Fc portion of IgG. Its mode of formation and pathologic action, if any, is unknown. In serum sickness, rubella, and viral hepatitis, there is a clear-cut temporal association with arthritic involvement. Interestingly, D. K. Onion, C. S. Crumpacter, and B. C. Gilliland report three cases of hepatitis in which arthritis and the presence of Australia antigen in circulation and in the synovial fluid preceded manifestations of clinical hepatitis and circulating antibodies. The findings suggest an immune complex, heteroimmune etiology for at least some forms of nonbacterial arthritis.

REFERENCES

Andres, G. A., Accini, L., Hsu, K. C., Zubriskie, J. B., and Seegal, B. C. Electron microscopic studies of human glomerulonephritis with ferritin-conjugated antibody. Localization of antigen-antibody complexes in glomerular structures of patients with acute glomerulonephritis. *J. Exp. Med.,* **123**:399, 1966.

Bucsi, R. A. and Strausser, H. R. The effect of neonatal thymectomy in the induction of experimental autoimmune thyroiditis in the rat. *Experientia,* **28**:194, 1972.

Cho, H. J. and Ingram, D. G. Antigen and antibody in Aleutian disease in mink. I. Precipitation reaction by agar gel electrophoresis. *J. Immunol.,* **108**:555, 1972.

Clarke, R. R. and Van de Velde, R. L. Congenital myasthenia gravis. *Am. J. Dis. Child.,* **122**:356, 1971.

Dixon, F. J. The pathogenesis of glomerulonephritis. *Am. J. Med.,* **44**:493, 1962.

Doniach, D., Walker, J. G., Riott, I. M., and Berg, P. A. "Autoallergic" hepatitis. *New Eng. J. Med.,* **282**:86, 1970.

Edgington, T. S. and Ritt, D. J. Intrahepatic expression of serum hepatitis virus-associated antigens. *J. Exp. Med.,* **134**:871, 1971.

Estes, D. and Christian, C. C. The natural history of systemic lupus erythematosus by prospective analysis. *Medicine,* **50**:85, 1971.

Fish, A. J., Herdman, R. C., Michael, A. F., Pickering, R. J., and Good, R. A. Epidemic acute glomerulonephritis associated with type 4g streptococcal pyoderma. II. Correlative study of light, immunofluorescent, and electron microscopic findings. *Am. J. Med.,* **48**:28, 1970.

Freedman, P., Meister, H. P., Lee, H. J., Smith, E. C., Co, B. S., and Nidus, P. D. The renal response to streptococcal infection. *Medicine,* **49**:433, 1970.

Fudenberg, H. H. Genetically determined immune deficiency as the predisposing cause of "autoimmunity" and lymphoid neoplasia. *Am. J. Med.,* **51**:295, 1971.

Germuth, F. G., Senterfit, L. B., and Dreesmen, G. R. Immune complex disease. V. The nature of the circulating complexes associated with glomerular alterations in the chronic BSA-rabbit system. *Johns Hopk. Med. J.,* **130**:344, 1972.

Guerra-Rodrigo, F. and Cardoso, J. P. M. Pemphigus vegetans. *Arch. Dermatol.,* **104**:411, 1971.

Gutman, R. A., Striker, G. E., Gilliland, B. C., and Cutler, R. E. The immune complex glomerulonephritis of bacterial endocarditis. *Medicine* **51**:1, 1972.

Henson, P. M. and Chochrane, C. G. Acute immune complex disease in rabbits. The role of complement and of a leukocyte-dependent release of vasoactive amines from platelets. *J. Exp. Med.,* **133**:554, 1971.

Jordan, R. E., Sams, W. M., Jr., Diaz, G., and Butner, E. H. Negative complement immunofluorescence in pemphigus. *J. Invest. Dermat.,* **57**:407, 1971.

Kaplan, E. L., Antony, B. F., Chapman, S. S., and Wannamaker, L. W. Epidemic acute glomerulonephritis associated with type 4g streptococcal pyodermia. I. Clinical and laboratory findings. *Am. J. Med.,* **48**:9, 1970.

Kraft, S. C., Rothberg, R. M., McCaffry, T. D., Jr., and Gelzayn, E. A. The intestinal immunologic system in inflammatory bowel disease. In "The secretory immunologic system," D. H. Dayton, Jr., P. A. Small, Jr., R. M. Chanovk, H. E. Kaufman, and T. B. Tomasi, Jr., eds. U.S. Government Printing Office, Washington, 1969.

Lerner, R. A., Glassrock, R. J., and Dixon, F. J. The role of antiglomerular basement membrane antibody in the pathogenesis of human glomerulonephritis. *J. Exp. Med.,* **126**:989, 1967.

Mattioli, M. and Reichlin, M. Characterization of a soluble nuclear ribonucleoprotein antigen reactive with SLE sera. *J. Immunol.,* **107**:1281, 1971.

McPhaul, J. J. and Dixon, F. J. Characterization of immunoglobulin G antiglomerular basement membrane antibodies eluted from kidneys of patients with glomerulonephritis. II. IgG subtypes and *in vitro* complement fixation. *J. Immunol.,* **107**:678, 1971.

Mellors, R. Leukemia virus and autoimmune disease of NZB mice. *Ann. N.Y. Acad. Sci.,* **183**:221, 1971.

Miescher, P. A. and Müller-Eberhard, H. J. "Textbook of immunopathology," Vols. I and II. Grune and Stratton, New York, 1967 and 1969.

Northway, J. D. and Tan, E. M. Differentiation of antinuclear antibodies giving speckled staining patterns in immunofluorescence. *Clin. Immunol. Immunobiol.,* 1:140, 1972.

Onion, D. K., Crumpacter, C. S., and Gilliland, B. C. Arthritis of hepatitis associated with Australia antigen. *Ann. Int. Med.,* **75**:29, 1971.

Pan, I. C., Tsai, K. S., and Karstad, L. Glomerulonephritis in Aleutian disease of mink: Histological and immunofluorescence studies. *J. Path.,* **101**:119, 1970.

Paul, W. E., Katz, P. H., and Benaceraff, B. Augmented anti-S_{111} antibody responses to an S_{111}-protein conjugate. *J. Immunol.*, **107**:685, 1971.

Perlo, V. P., Arnason, B., Poskanzer, D., Castleman, B., Schwab, R. S., Osserman, D. E., Papatestis, A., Alpert, L. and Kark, A. The role of thymectomy in the treatment of myasthenia gravis. *Ann. N.Y. Acad. Sci.*, **183**, 308, 1971.

Poskitt, T. R. Immunologic and electron microscopic studies in Goodpasture's syndrome. *Am. J. Med.*, **49**:250, 1970.

Proskitt, A. J., Weatherbee, L., Easterling, R. E., Greene, J. A., and Wella, J. M. Goodpasture's syndrome. A report of five cases and review of the literature. *Am. J. Med.*, **48**:162, 1970.

Rowland, L. P. Immunosuppressive drugs in the treatment of myasthenia gravis. *Ann. N.Y. Acad. Sci.*, **183**:351, 1971.

Sherlock, S. The immunology of liver disease. *Am. J. Med.*, **49**:693, 1970.

Shirisinha, S. and Eisen, H. N. Autoimmune-like antibodies to the ligand binding site of myeloma proteins. *Proc. Nat. Acad. Sci. U.S.*, **68**:3130, 1971.

Silverman, D. A. and Rose, N. R. Autoimmunity in methylcholanthrene-induced and spontaneous thyroiditis in buffalo strain rats. *Proc. Soc. Exp. Biol. Med.*, **138**:579, 1971.

Tan, E. M. and Lerner, R. A. An immunological approach to the fate of nuclear and nucleolar macromolecules during the cell cycle. *J. Mol. Biol.*, **68**:107, 1972.

Index

239